More Praise For *Politically Incorrect Nutrition*

Politically Incorrect Nutrition is a book that dares to challenge the prevailing mythology of food and drink. After reading Michael Barbee's compelling book, you'll never again take for granted that your fluoridated water, soy foods, aspartame, or green tea are as safe as their proponents claim. A must-read for anyone who is concerned that the media and medical establishment aren't giving the entire picture of nutrition today.

Mary J. Shomon
Living Well With Hypothyroidism,
Living Well With Autoimmune Disease, and
What Your Doctor May Not Tell You About Parkinson's Disease

Michael Barbee's well-researched and engaging exposé of both the myths regarding our most popular and unpopular foods and some of our most entrenched health assumptions, is a must-read. We are very fortunate to be given access to these vital facts before we have unknowingly exposed our children and ourselves to further culinary dangers.

Julia Ross, MA,
The Mood Cure and the best-seller, *The Diet Cure*

Nowadays it is up to the patient to do his homework before making decisions. This excellent guide will help anyone sort through all the options before making a decision.

Joanie Greggains, fitness expert
KGO Radio and syndicated TV show, *Morning Stretch*

The information in *Politically Incorrect Nutrition* is right on the money. It is current, cutting-edge, and very much on target. This is a book I can highly recommend for each and every one of us.

Ann Louise Gittleman, Ph.D.
New York Times Bestseller, *The Fat Flush Plan*

POLITICALLY INCORRECT NUTRITION

*Finding Reality in the Mire of
Food Industry Propaganda*

by

Michael Barbee

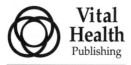

Vital
Health
Publishing

Ridgefield, CT

Politically Incorrect Nutrition: Finding Reality in the Mire of
Food Industry Propaganda

Copyright © 2004, Michael Barbee

Book Design: cover, OnThe Dot Designs; interior, Cathy Lombardi

Published by: Vital Health Publishing
                  P.O. Box 152
                  Ridgefield, CT 06877
                  Website: www.vitalhealthbooks.com
                  E-mail: info@vitalhealthbooks.com
                  Phone: 203-894-1882
                  Orders: 1-877-VIT-BOOK

Printed in the United States of America
ISBN: 978-1-890612-34-4

This book is dedicated to my father, Delbert Barbee.
He knew to question what was commonly believed to be true.
He told me over thirty years ago that eating margarine was
no better than eating plastic. He knew the value of whole, natural foods.

Acknowledgments

I wish to thank Andreas Schuld, Dick and Valerie James, Betty Martini, Dr. Mary Enig, and Sally Fallon of the Weston A. Price Foundation for the wonderful research they have done—and for their answers to my many questions.

Thanks also to Nutrition Consultant Becky Saala for having introduced me to the good folks at the Institute for Educational Therapy (IET) in Cotati, California—a holistic vocational school offering professional certification in nutrition and the culinary arts.

And thanks to my wife, Sharon, for her suggestions and her advice to temper my comments about the "diet dictocrats" so that my displeasure with them would not act to harangue the reader. I hope she was successful.

Table of Contents

Preface

Eating for health is both a science and an art. Researchers continually update our knowledge about the science of nutrition, about how the body responds biochemically to the substances we ingest. Almost daily, it seems, we are bombarded with new information about diets, much of it contradicting what we have long held as true. Should we eat fewer carbohydrates or more? More protein? Or more "healthy" fats?

There is much confusion in the minds of many. And much fear. We have been told that a great number of cancers can be directly tied to the foods we eat—or don't eat. We want to be healthy. We want to do the right thing, but the overload of information and advice is causing many simply to throw up their hands in disgust, despair, or resignation.

In the process, the art of eating is becoming a lost one. I'm not talking about gourmet eating here, but rather the intuitive art or ability to listen to the body—to be conscious of our bodies' responses to what we put in our mouths—to be aware of what foods truly nourish us.

It is easy to see the signs of a public out of tune with food: high rates of heart disease, osteoporosis, cancer, and the almost epidemic rates of obesity, diabetes, and hypothyroidism. If we continue to hide our heads in the sand about nutrition, or on the other hand, if we quickly jump on any new diet bandwagon without giving a close look at the science behind it, we will continue to fight a losing battle.

While the science of nutrition constantly changes, there is one science that does not change, one science that is often at odds with the nutritional health of the nation: political science. Sadly, it seems, the prime motivation of many politicians is to keep power, and to do so they often form an unhealthy partnership with corporate interests. In an attempt to make profits, industry enlists the aid of elected officials and their appointed bureaucrats to make policy which affects public health.

This is no surprise, I'm sure. This is not news. But the extent to which the safety of what we eat and drink is affected by corporate influence and greed may come as a surprise. In fact, we should be outraged. Our health is at stake as we are poisoned daily with what should never be in our foods, and we are also poisoned with bad advice. Some of that advice is well-intentioned, but much of it is based on old, unscientific information. Some of it is based on myth. And some of that information is actually *misinformation* designed to keep the public ignorant while the food companies reap enormous profits.

This book makes no attempt, as in a court trial, to present both sides of nutritional controversies. With certain issues, there are many studies that arrive at quite opposite conclusions. Agribusiness, factory farms, and industrial and political concerns have already presented their case. With faulty or falsified research, with a misinterpretation of the facts, they have greatly influenced what we consume. As a consequence, the health of the nation has suffered. It is time to present the other side. It's time to show how we have been misled. The readers can act as the jury, using common sense to arrive at a better understanding of nutrition. The readers can determine whether the information presented here rings true in their own lives on both an intellectual and an intuitive level.

There is a battle of immense significance taking place today, the outcome of which will affect the health of everyone in this county. On one side we have the science of nutrition and the art of eating. On the other side, the opponent is represented by the science of politics and the art of making money. Let's clear the air and see what the facts are.

GREEN TEA

Propaganda: Drink 3–6 cups of green tea a day for its antioxidants.

Reality: Today's cup of green tea is often contaminated with unprecedented amounts of fluoride, aluminum, and DDT, and regular consumption can lead to serious health problems.

A CUP OF CONTAMINANTS

Our society has always been quick to seize upon the latest fads, whether they're old ones like hula hoops, pet rocks, and beanie babies, or newer ones that are not likely to go away any time soon like SUVs, cell phones, and three-dollar cups of coffee. No one wants to be left behind. The same is true when it comes to dietary health: the hottest new food or supplement, guaranteed to provide longevity, quickly floods the market. For instance, have you noticed all the flavors and brands of green tea available today? Green tea is catching on in a big way. In the United States the wholesale value of green tea has jumped from $2 million to over $25 million in the last ten years.

Some health fads that are based on *good science*, like the increasing use of certain antioxidant supplements, seem to be of considerable benefit for many nutrient-deprived Americans. The use of green tea as an aid to health, on the other hand, may prove to be a disaster.

Green tea (and black tea, which comes from the same plant) have been used for centuries for their health-promoting qualities. Recently, special attention has been paid to the antioxidant nature of green tea's polyphenols. There is reasonable evidence to suggest that these antioxidant chemicals (catechins, in particular) may offer some protection against cancer and heart disease.

The problem is that today's green tea is not the same as it was hundreds of years ago. The plant is the same. The polyphenols are there. But there is also something else in today's green tea in quantities that are unprecedented and quite troublesome: fluoride.

TOO MUCH OF A "GOOD" THING

The tea plant (*Camellia sinensis*) absorbs and stores more fluoride than any other plant. Those who market green tea claim this is a good thing. The more fluoride the better, they say. You get fewer cavities, they say, along with the cancer-fighting properties of the tea. A growing number of scientists, however, are coming to the conclusion that fluoride is, among other things, a cancer promoter.

Despite what many nutrition texts tell us, fluoride has no recognized, essential use in the human body.[1] It is simply a poisonous substance—one of the most toxic known to man. What's more, green tea is becoming increasingly more contaminated with fluoride than ever before because of the use of fluoride-containing pesticides and fertilizers. Unfortunately, as a result of widespread water, soil, and air pollution from phosphate fertilizer plants, even organic green tea cannot always escape increasing contamination. A comparison could be made between modern green tea and much of the fish consumed today, which is often tainted with dangerous levels of mercury. Historically, both fish and green tea were positive influences on health when they were uncontaminated. Sadly, some health experts have been forced to recommend the avoidance of all fish and instead suggest we derive its benefits from mercury-free cod liver oil.

If fluoride is such a toxic contaminant, then why are we adding this stuff to our water in an attempt to improve dental health? Scientists at the Environmental Protection Agency (EPA) would like to know this as well. Not long ago they called for a moratorium on water fluoridation. Unfortunately, they are not the ones who make public policy. They do know, however, that fluoride increases the body's ability to store aluminum in various organs, including the brain. And much of the fluoride that finds its way into green tea is aluminum fluoride. This raises real concerns about the role fluoride and aluminum play in the development of Alzheimer's disease.[2,3] (See the chapter titled "Fluoridation.")

But how much fluoride could there possibly be in a cup of green tea? It depends, of course, on where and how it was grown. At the low end, some teas show about 1 mg in one cup of tea, the same amount one would find in an entire quart of artificially fluoridated water. Other studies have shown that in various parts of the world the daily intakes of fluoride from tea alone are about 4-9 mg per day, depending on how many cups are consumed.[4-6] And here's a good one: one sample of Chinese green tea recently analyzed had a whopping 22 mg of fluoride per tea bag.[7]

EXCEEDING THE "SAFE" LIMIT

To put all this into perspective, it is important to know that most teas evaluated exceed the maximum fluoride contaminant level of 4 parts per million set by the EPA for drinking water. Any person with a lifetime of consuming more than the established contaminant level is expected to develop crippling skeletal fluorosis (denser, but more brittle bones). The first stage of this disease—vague muscular pains, as well as sporadic pain and stiffness in the joints and spine—is estimated to develop in as little as five years, based on the daily consumption of the amount of fluoride found in three or four average cups of green tea.[8] This early stage of fluorosis is not well studied or understood in this country and may be misdiagnosed as rheumatoid or osteoarthritis.[9-11] It should be noted that Hawaii is the least fluoridated state and has the least number of arthritic adults.[12] In terms of total fluoride intake, don't forget about the fluoride accumulating in the body from sources other than tea: water, toothpaste, rinses, pesticides, soft drinks, and foods processed with fluoridated water. There's more in your can of Coke than sugar and caffeine.

Another problem associated with fluoride consumption is the impact it has on the thyroid. Fluoride suppresses thyroid function, leading to *hypothyroidism*. In fact, many years ago fluoride was used as a means to treat *hyperthyroidism*, in amounts less than what can be found in a cup of many green teas.[13] Furthermore, in populations where there is high consumption of green tea, like the Japanese, there is a much higher incidence of thyroid cancer.[14] One supplier of organic green tea has recommended that its product not be consumed by people taking the thyroid medication Synthroid™ because the fluoride content of its tea would interfere with the effect of this drug.

Just as the increasing incidence of Alzheimer's disease parallels the increasing consumption of fluoride during the last forty to fifty years, the symptoms and associations of hypothyroidism show an increasing prevalence in our society: carpal tunnel syndrome, loss of libido, arthritis, lupus, fibromyalgia, and weight gain. Preventative medicine expert Dr. Stephen Langer suggests that as much as 40 percent of the population may have subclinical hypothyroidism, a condition not detected by traditional blood chemistry work.[15] The fluoride that pervades our food and water supply must surely be considered a culprit, with tea drinkers at higher risk.

A CUP OF DDT

To make matters worse, some samples of green tea recently analyzed were contaminated with DDT and the DDT-like pesticide Dursban—raising concerns about tea's possible role in the development of breast cancer.[16] DDT was banned in the United States in 1972, and Dursban has just recently been banned for household use. India and China, however, continue to produce DDT, which is used in over two dozen third-world nations, finding its way into some tea leaves in small amounts.

With all this bad news, it seems that the antioxidants that tea drinkers are hoping to acquire from their beverage may come, ironically, at the expense of their overall health. There is even some evidence to show that fluoride actually inhibits the beneficial aspects of antioxidants.[17] It seems much wiser and safer, then, to obtain free-radical scavenging antioxidants from food sources like fruits and vegetables or from the well-studied supplements like vitamins C and E, zinc, selenium, CoQ10, and N-Acetyl Cysteine (NAC)—even perhaps a bit of chocolate.

Chocolate has four times the amount of antioxidant catechins as green tea.[18, 19] Significant amounts of these health-promoting substances can be found as well in red wine, apples, and pears. Some studies have found that the catechins contained in green tea do not help to combat factors related to heart disease.[20, 21] Other studies found that those in chocolate could protect the heart, as well as helping to regulate the immune system.[22] Another study showed that the catechins in apples and wine proved beneficial, but not those in tea.[23] Research on the effects of green tea has been quite mixed, to say the least.

Looking at the Studies

It is essential to read the results of research carefully. One of America's best known health and nutrition writers recently promoted the consumption of three to six cups of tea a day, citing research showing that animals drinking green tea instead of water reduced their incidence of arthritis. What she failed to point out is that the animals did not actually consume tea, but rather, they drank water spiked with the isolated antioxidants that can be found in tea.[24] Other studies show good results from antioxidant extracts of green tea without the test animals actually consuming the whole beverage, replete with its fluoride arsenal—but tea gets the credit. Very misleading.

Research from Taiwan in 1990 found green tea consumption was linked to higher rates of stomach cancer.[25] Conversely, and getting a lot of press recently, is a 2001 study from UCLA involving 732 individuals that showed drinking green tea appeared to reduce rates of stomach cancer in China, which has the highest stomach cancer rate in the world.[26] Researchers speculate that it may be the antioxidants in the tea that are responsible for less stomach cancer in tea drinkers. They are not certain.

Fluoride—Cure or Cause?

Surely, fluoride's role in stomach cancer must be considered. Fluoride is known to be toxic to bacteria. Since some stomach cancers have been tied to the *H. pylori* bacterium—the same one linked to ulcers, it is possible that the fluoride in tea kills off this bacterium if enough tea is consumed. This, however, still leaves the door open for fluoride's cancer-promoting properties to result in stomach cancers not related to *H. pylori* —as well as in thousands of other deaths from cancer in general (see the "Fluoridation" chapter).

The lead researcher of a stomach cancer study at UCLA, Dr. Zhang, was contacted by the author of this book about the possible role of fluoride in *H. pylori*-induced stomach cancer. He replied that it is something that should be studied.

Dr. Zhang, however, may not have to bother. Another 2001 study—a much larger one involving 26,000 people—found no association between green tea consumption and the risk of gastric cancer.[27] In 2002 an even larger study of 73,000 individuals found the same thing.[28] For some reason these studies don't get much press coverage.

What We Don't Hear

In the haste to profit from the public's desire to jump on the newest health bandwagon, we usually hear only about the good health of populations consuming green tea. What we don't hear about, like the studies noted above that show *positive* effects of green tea consumption, is the research that shows those getting the greatest amounts of catechins from tea may also consume more fiber and vitamins A and C.[29] We also don't hear about studies that show green tea is *not* helpful as a cancer preventative[30]— or those showing a possible increased risk of cancer (rectal) from consuming green tea,[31] or studies showing a positive correlation between higher intakes of tea and increased rates of colon cancer.[32, 33]

We are further told that drinking green tea may lessen the chances of developing osteoporosis, which unfortunately is defined by many people simply in terms of bone density. Fluoride consumption, as in tea, does indeed create denser bones. However, this increased bone mineral density (BMD) comes at a stiff price. The bones become more brittle and are more prone to fracture. And bone strength is reduced.[34] As mentioned, arthritic symptoms are also associated with high fluoride intake. Many people have reported that their arthritis vanished after eliminating tea from their diets.

Since most Americans daily consume, from multiple sources, more fluoride than what is deemed to be safe by the EPA, it would be ill-advised to intentionally add more of this stuff to the diet in the form of tea. It becomes apparent that consuming three to six cups of green tea a day, as recommended by some nutrition experts, is likely to lead to serious health problems in a few short years because of its fluoride, aluminum, and possible DDT contamination. As far as a choice of beverages is concerned, herbal teas taste better. So does chocolate.

■■ **TIPS:** ■■

For antioxidants: consume fresh, organic fruits and vegetables, and/or supplement with vitamins C and E, selenium, CoQ10, and N-Acetyl Cysteine.

Great news! Dark chocolate (organic) has four times the amount of antioxidants as green tea per serving! Look for dark chocolate, which contains at least 70% cocoa solids.

Soy

Propaganda: Soy protects against breast cancer and osteoporosis—
so, like the Asians, we should eat more tofu and other soy products.

Reality: The Asian diet is not soy based. Unfermented soy products
are not digestible. Soy is not a complete protein, and a pesticide-
laden, soy-based diet can lead to severe nutritional deficiencies and
hormonal imbalances.

No Wonder Food

The recent consumer interest in soy products has probably made happy
campers out of Monsanto and food giant Archer Daniels Midland. Monsanto can sell more of its genetically altered seeds, which can tolerate
greater amounts of another of their products (Round-Up™), and Archer
Daniels Midland can sell its beans and processed soy goods hand-over-
bushel to countless businesses. With food aisles today brimming with
over 300 soy products, including soy protein supplements, soy breakfast
cereals, soy energy bars, and an endless array of soy beverages made from
these beans, is soy beer soon to follow? Yes, in fact it's already here.

We are told over and over how soy is a wonder food—how it protects
humans from practically all known diseases, particularly breast cancer and
osteoporosis. The Japanese, we are informed, consume huge amounts of
soy and have low rates of these diseases relative to Western populations.
So, eat soy and live a long, healthy life.

But how much is fact and how much is hype? How much of what the
media tells us is based on good, impartial science, and how much is based
on the premise that a lie, often repeated, eventually is accepted as the truth?

First of all, according to a recent evaluation of the existing evidence,
consuming large amounts of soy cannot be directly tied to lowered rates
of breast cancer and heart disease—or even to less osteoporosis and fewer
unpleasant postmenopausal symptoms.[1] There could be any number of
factors involved in the Japanese diet that make them less susceptible to
these conditions. It could be due to the health-generating effects of
tighter social bonds, which their population often exhibits. It could be
that a lack of American-style junk food in their diet results in better
health—or maybe a heavy consumption of fish soup along with meals
that typically consist of thirty or more varied ingredients is healthful. We
just don't know for certain, although there is evidence that consumption
of sea vegetables, with their high iodine content, may result in lowered
rates of breast cancer in Japan.[2] It should not be forgotten that, although
the Japanese diet in general appears to be healthier than a typical American

diet, the Japanese suffer from high rates of esophagus, stomach, pancreas, liver, and thyroid cancers. Soy appears to offer no protection here.

What is more interesting, however, is the fact that it is simply a myth that Asians eat a "soy-based diet." One survey has shown that a typical intake of soy amounts to about two teaspoons a day in China.[3] Another study indicates the intake is less than one serving (1/4 cup) of soy every day or two in Japan.[4] They are not gobbling up the soy milk and tofu as we have been led to believe. *But we are.* And there may be some negative health consequences as a result of loading up on soy products. We have heard plenty in the press about the value of soy products, especially soy isoflavones. Some research attests to the value of these phytoestrogens. Many recent studies, however, reveal the opposite. But because the soy industry is such big business today, much of the negative press about soy is slow to appear. For example, little mention was made of the conclusions arrived at by a researcher who warned against the wide use of soy isoflavones: "Recent studies have finally indicated a potential role for soy isoflavones in inducing chromosomal changes in cells exposed *in vitro* (in a test tube) and potentiating chemical carcinogens."[5]

In other words, the jury is still out. There is still much to be learned about soy's effects on living systems. Caution is called for, particularly in view of the fact that, according to researcher Mary Enig, Ph.D., there has been so much demand for soy oil that the leftover soy protein needed to find a market. Since animals don't tolerate it very well, the new market has become us. Are we being misled about soy's benefits? There is still much speculation about the role of soy in human health. But it is speculation that deserves to be taken seriously. The American public has bought into the concept that soy is a miracle food—the more the better. Unfortunately, it appears that the public is being subjected to a huge soy experiment that could lead to dire consequences. It's time to take a look at some information about soy that we don't see in the popular magazines.

A PLANT POISON

Much attention, of course, has been given to the power of soy isoflavones. These are estrogens produced by the plant in order to protect itself from attack by hungry creatures. Some plants evolved to employ thorns, bitter-tasting substances, or even toxins, to thwart invaders and thus survive.

The soy plant, however, employs a different tactic. It developed a plant estrogen that, when repeatedly devoured by a mammalian pest, would result in hormonal changes to the predator, interrupting its reproductive cycle. How sneaky!

This might seem far-fetched, but consider the fact that we are plant predators, too, and it is quite possible that our hormonal balance and reproductive health is negatively impacted by consuming soy isoflavones. It is believed that many years ago, soy was not considered an edible crop. It was used in plant-rotation practices to impart nitrogen to the soil. Did earlier societies know something we don't? Perhaps.

However, there are some Asian celibate monks today who use soy foods to dampen their libido.[6] Apparently this is more popular than taking a cold shower. Japanese wives are said to slip their husbands extra tofu when the man's sexual appetite becomes too much to bear[7]—the Japanese version of, "Not tonight, honey; I have a headache."

Researchers once commonly considered the effects of soy isoflavones to be antiestrogenic—a good thing—helping to prevent cancer. In other words, soy isoflavones can block estrogen cell receptors. Some researchers, however, now assert that these dietary estrogens (genistein, in particular) can also stimulate the estrogen receptors, thereby setting off an entire chain of hormonal events. It is possible that soy isoflavones can behave like a dangerous chemical xenoestrogen—such as DDT. Dr. Craig Dees of Oak Ridge National Laboratory has found that soy isoflavones cause breast cancer cells to grow. In the lab genistein has been found to enhance the proliferation of estrogen-dependent human breast cancer cells.[8] Some plant estrogens can act as weak estrogens, which may be good, or they may do the opposite. Some appear to be estrogen-mimics that carry a powerful punch, causing researchers to regard isoflavones as "a double-edged sword."[9] Others have even claimed that there is no direct evidence for the beneficial effects of phytoestrogens in humans, stating that "it is plausible the phytoestrogens, as any exogenous hormonally active agent, might cause adverse effects in the endocrine system, i.e., act as endocrine (hormone) disrupters."[10] Incidentally, use of Monsanto's Round-Up™ on their variety of soybeans is reported to increase the amount of these isoflavones. These beans account for half of the soybeans grown in this country.

SOY AND EARLY PUBERTY

Some of soy's hormonal effects appear to be taking their toll on children. "Young children are especially susceptible to elevated levels of estrogen. Thus, there is a clear and serious health issue at hand," claims geneticist Dr. Ricarda Steinbrecher.[11] Besides causing zinc deficiency in infants, the increased use of soy formula is suspected as a leading cause of increased rates of premature sexual development; children are entering puberty much earlier than normal. According to environmental toxicologist Mike Fitzpatrick, the exclusive use of soy infant formula is the equivalent of consuming one or two birth control pills daily, on an estrogenic basis.[12]

Soy infant formulas provide six to eleven times more isoflavones per body weight than the dose needed to create hormonal effects in adults consuming soy (two glasses of soy milk per day). Such an amount changes menstrual patterns in women.[13] What is the equivalent amount of soy doing to children? Youngsters consuming soy formula seem to show a greater tendency toward developing autoimmune thyroid disease,[14] as well as diabetes.[15] It is possible that soy-fed infants are developing thymic and immune abnormalities as well.[16] For these reasons, Switzerland, England, Australia, and New Zealand recommend medically monitored use of soy for babies and pregnant women.

Recently, a team of researchers at Lehigh University in Pennsylvania found that soy isoflavones fed to rodents significantly accelerated the onset of puberty. The leader of the team, Professor of Biology Jill Schneider, says that isoflavones, which bind to estrogen receptors and can mimic this hormone, might be linked to a number of health risks, including breast cancer and accelerated aging in the brain. She adds that investigators have asked the Food and Drug Administration (FDA) not to allow soy manufacturers to claim their products are good for health.[17]

Even consumption of soy by the pregnant mother has its risks. According to two senior scientists at the FDA (Doerge and Sheehan), who refused to rubber-stamp the approval of soy isoflavones as GRAS (generally recognized as safe), ". . . consumption of isoflavones during pregnancy in humans could be a risk factor for normal brain and reproductive tract development."[18]

Tampering with young children's hormones by adding soy to their diets is also thought to impair mental growth as well, leading to learning disabilities, which are widespread today. Add to this the fact that liquid soy products, often produced in aluminum tanks, contain 50 to 100 times more aluminum than breast milk (in addition to high levels of cadmium), and you have a situation where babies are put at risk of aluminum toxicity and its impact on the developing brain. The high manganese content of soy formula has already been implicated in harming the infant brain.

THE THYROID AT RISK

Some researchers state flat-out that soy isoflavones are a form of medication. As with most drugs, there are good and there are bad aspects. The *positive effects* must be weighed against the *side effects*. Menopausal, "estrogen-deficient" women are thought to derive some relief from hot flashes and other ailments by consuming soy isoflavones. Although the research is mixed, particularly with regard to the reduction of hot flashes, these apparent benefits are being called into question.[19] The British government's Committee on Toxicity in Foods (COT) recently released their assessment of soy products and isoflavone supplements (Oct. 2002). After analyzing this long report, soy expert Valerie James notes the following: "As for claims that these products improve hormonal balance, prevent prostate cancers, prevent heart disease, stop osteoporosis and improve brain function, the COT found no proof of any of this."[20]

As for using soy to treat menopausal symptoms, COT's chapter on hormonal effects states: "The weight of evidence does not strongly support the view that supplementation of the diet with soy or isoflavones alleviates menopausal symptoms."[21] Women who continue to use these products to achieve a greater level of comfort may find, however, that what they are seeking may come at a great cost—*hypothyroidism.*

It is believed by a number of health educators that the United States is experiencing a hypothyroid epidemic. In fact, we are already seeing increased signs of general fatigue, weakness, constipation, depression, and weight gain—signs of an underactive thyroid. Suppression of this gland has been shown to develop with eating as little as two tablespoons of soybeans per day.[22]

It has been known for over fifty years that soy has a negative impact on the thyroid. Research in Japan concluded that in humans a daily intake of 30 grams of soybeans (1 ounce) over the course of three months caused enlargement of the thyroid, as well as suppressed thyroid function. Some subjects even developed goiter. The subjects returned to normal when the soy was discontinued.[23] One of the isoflavones involved with this process, genistein, inhibits thyroid function more effectively than medication given to control hyperthyroidism.

Fluoride also suppresses thyroid function. Its consumption from all sources has risen steadily over the last few decades. When this fact is coupled with statistics that show sales of soy milk in the United States rising from $2 million in 1980 to over $300 million today, it is likely that the hypothyroid epidemic is a greater problem than most of us can imagine. It is estimated that at least 10 percent of the population has an underactive thyroid, and more than 12 million Americans may be walking around with their problem undiagnosed.

SOY PROTEIN NOT PERFECT

As noted, soy isoflavones were not granted GRAS status by the FDA. Archer Daniels Midland withdrew their request before action could be taken after a large number of studies poured in relating to soy dangers, not the least of which was concern about toxins and carcinogens that are formed during soy processing. The FDA did, however, allow soy products to carry labels stating that the consumption of soy protein is heart-healthy. Soy protein does indeed lower total cholesterol levels, but it may do so at the expense of lowering beneficial HDL cholesterol, according to some research.[24]

Some additional points need to be made about soy protein. First, contrary to what some people believe, *soy is not a complete protein.* It is deficient in the important amino acids methionine and cystine; the promotion of tissue growth and of general health suffers as a consequence. Soy protein is difficult to digest because it contains substantial amounts of trypsin inhibitors, which interfere with protein digestion and can lead to pancreatic disorders.[25] Vegetarians who rely largely on soy for their protein source may not be getting as much as they need—and may be getting an inferior protein at that. When protein digestion is hampered, the pancreas must work harder. It often becomes enlarged and more subject to cancer.

Again, in Asia soy consumption is not as high as we are commonly led to believe. In China, protein from pork and grains far outweighs that obtained from soy and all other legumes combined, and for the Japanese, fish provides the most protein. Incidentally, in terms of cancer, according to nutritionist and author Robert Crayhon: "Animal studies suggest that whey and meat protein are much more protective against cancer than soy protein."[26]

Furthermore, the vitamin B_{12} compound found in plant sources cannot be absorbed by the body, and according to researchers Mary Enig and Sally Fallon, modern soy products increase the body's requirement for vitamin B_{12}.[27] This is bad news for strict vegetarians who rely on soy for their protein. Since they do not consume animal products, which are the best source for B_{12}, they can develop a deficiency in this essential nutrient.

In addition, if soy consumption reduces beneficial HDL cholesterol as well as overall cholesterol, this could be more than a mere trade-off. In fact, researchers have concluded that soy milk (powdered) significantly increases a substance in the blood called LP(a), which is a strong marker for increased risk of heart disease. The authors of the study suggested that such soy milk should be excluded from the diet.[28] For those who still feel that soy protects the heart (as advertisers are allowed to say), the amount of soy protein (at least 25 grams) recommended by the FDA to reduce cholesterol contains significantly more isoflavones than the amounts found to induce hypothyroid conditions in human subjects.[29] The recommended 25 grams is considerably higher than the typical daily Japanese soy protein intake of 7–8 grams.[30] People particularly susceptible to an impaired thyroid gland appear to be the elderly and women in transitional menopause. These groups are often the targets for soy marketing. It should be noted that an underactive thyroid is another risk factor for heart disease. Also, pregnant women with underactive thyroids that are not treated have been shown to be four times more likely to give birth to children with low IQs.[31]

Monkey Business at the FDA

Finally, approval of health claims by the FDA often has a price tag. If you have the money and the influence, you can frequently get what you want. The large soy industry has both. *U.S.A. Today* (Sept. 25, 2000) reported that since 1998 at least 92 percent of FDA approval committee meetings had at least one member with a conflict of interest. In 55 percent of the meetings, at least half of the FDA advisors who were consulted had a conflict. Federal law prohibits this kind of financial conflict, but since 1998 the FDA has lifted the restrictions over 800 times. What is more appalling is the fact that the FDA keeps these conflict-of-interest dealings secret, making it impossible to track the money and the influence.

Apparently the wine industry does not have the clout (or money) to match that of the giant soy concerns in influencing government policy. Otherwise, their desire to put health claims on their product would have been successful because wine's link to heart health is better documented than soy's claims.

More Soy Problems

Another claim we hear often is that soy may be useful in combating osteoporosis. This appears unlikely since soy products can cause deficiencies in both calcium and vitamin D.[32] As further evidence, a recent study found that soy foods do not contribute to greater bone density in humans.[33] In addition, concentrations of oxalate, a compound contained in most soy products, are so high that this calcium-binding substance is a danger to those with a tendency to develop kidney stones. Researchers concluded that no soy food tested could be recommended to patients with a personal history of kidney stones.[34]

Soy consumption may contribute to other deficiencies as well. Soy contains substantial amounts of phytic acid (phytates). These substances, though valuable in small amounts, prevent the absorption of a number of minerals besides calcium—notably zinc, a nutrient in which a great number of Americans are deficient. An adequate supply of zinc is particularly important for brain health and for men's sexual health. Other legumes and grains contain phytic acid which, as a fiber, plays an important role in our health. But soy is especially high in this mineral-binding substance, and when soy is consumed in excess, problems are likely to arise.

IS YOUR SOY FERMENTED?

As mentioned earlier, the ancient Chinese initially did not use soy as a food crop. Eventually, they discovered that by fermenting the beans the soy protein could be digested more easily, and the phytic acid, toxins, and antinutrients would be largely destroyed. Therefore, tempeh, tamari (soy sauce), and natto became useful foods in small amounts. Natto is a pungent, fermented soy dish that is rich not only in beneficial bacteria, but also contains plenty of PQQ (Pyrroloquinoline quinone), a very recently discovered vitamin. PQQ is the first new vitamin discovered since 1948; it appears to support fertility. In addition, a landmark study of 143,000 Japanese women, which appeared to show that the incidence of breast cancer was reduced with soy, was based on the consumption of miso—another fermented product.[35]

There are anticarcinogenic substances found in soy that has been fermented—aglycones. In modern, nonfermented soy foods like tofu and soy milk, these aglycones exist in a different form and do not have anticancerous effects.[36] A more recent study looking at soy and breast cancer concluded, however, that there was no significant relationship between this disease and soy consumption.[37] But if one looks at the results of this study carefully, it can be seen that eating higher amounts of miso soup (five or more times a week) slightly reduced the incidence of breast cancer, whereas consuming higher amounts of tofu slightly increased breast cancer rates.

Today, however, what are we devouring in this country? Unfermented soy products—tofu and soy milk and "energy bars," which are usually loaded with soy isoflavones. Not only do these products retain much of the harmful substances of raw soy, but the processing of the beans to make such products as milk, tofu, and hydrolyzed vegetable protein adds potential carcinogens (3-MCPD and lysinoalanine) and other dangerous elements like aluminum, as noted earlier. This processing of nonfermented soy (milk, tofu) also appears to negate anticancer effects of soy substances and may even promote the development of breast cancer, according to some experts.

And just when you thought it couldn't get any worse—it does: A recent and well-designed study of older men of Japanese descent living in Hawaii found that consumption of tofu (two or more servings a week during midlife) appeared to be linked to the development of dementia.[38] What's not clear, however, is the exact mechanism—how tofu can cause cognitive impairment and brain atrophy in these men, conditions in which other factors were ruled out.

Could it be that the soy isoflavones disrupt the hormonal balance necessary to maintain brain health, as the researchers postulate? Perhaps it's a zinc depletion resulting from the phytic acid in tofu that causes changes in the brain in men already marginally low in this nutrient. Or maybe it's the aluminum content of the tofu. A combination of factors seems likely to result in a condition in which one researcher claimed that the brains of the tofu eaters seemed five years older than what they should have been. Certainly, more studies will need to follow this one. But, in the meantime, tofu, anyone?

I think I'll have the fermented soy instead, please. I'll stick to the traditional foods—not concentrated soy protein isolated, or modern tofu that is processed using harmful high temperatures. Miso and tempeh, please. And make them organic. But only a little bit, now and then. These fermented soy foods have a place in the diet. They are used frequently in Asia—in small amounts (usually as condiments)—not as a main course. We Americans love excess. A little common sense concerning soy is in order.

■■ TIPS: ■■

Use fermented soy products like tempeh, tamari, miso, and natto. These may have anticancerous effects. They can be found at health food stores.

Avoid soy milk, soy energy bars, hydrolyzed vegetable protein, and regular consumption of tofu.

CHOLESTEROL

Propaganda: Scientists find that feeding lots of cholesterol to bunnies (vegetarians) causes death. From this they conclude that dietary cholesterol causes death in humans.

Reality: Dietary cholesterol plays only a small part in overall cholesterol levels and is necessary for mental and physical human health. The *trans*-fat-filled, hydrogenated vegetable oils peddled by the food industry have been implicated in higher risks of both heart disease and cancer.

SOME GOOD NEWS

The year 1924 proved to be a disaster for the science of nutrition. That year, scientists fed lots of cholesterol to bunnies whose arteries got clogged, and they died. Conclusion: Feed people lots of cholesterol and they will die. Terrific science, except for a couple of things. The cholesterol fed to the rabbits was already damaged (oxidized—not fresh), and rabbits have very different digestive systems from humans. They are vegetarians and have no way of dealing with dietary cholesterol. But the news was out and the vegetable oil industry took note: "Scare the people about the cholesterol in animal fat and we'll sell them our vegetable fat."

Years later this deception was heightened by health experts who told us we would drop dead from heart attacks if we ate too many animal products. Didn't they check the facts? Didn't they see that in the early part of the twentieth century—when heart disease was practically unheard of—83 percent of the total fat intake came from animal fat?[1] Compare that to about 58 percent today—when heart disease is rampant.

Cholesterol (an alcohol, not a fat) is not the villain it is portrayed to be. We need it to keep our cells healthy, to help create the sex hormones, and to make sure the brain and nervous system function properly. Cholesterol is an important component of every cell. If we don't get enough in the diet, the body will make more. In fact, the liver acts like a cholesterol thermostat, controlling how much is in the bloodstream at a given time. Dietary cholesterol plays a relatively small part in overall blood cholesterol levels. In fact, our bodies *make three times more cholesterol than we typically eat.* But the general population has been led to believe that arteries will clog merely by looking at an egg. What has largely been hidden is the fact that, if for some reason there is not enough cholesterol supplied to the brain, those unfortunate people are more likely to suffer depression, exhibit aggressive behavior, and have higher suicide rates.[2-5]

Very low cholesterol levels are indeed dangerous. Low cholesterol levels are equated with a greater risk of dying from cancer.[6,7] Our fear of the cholesterol found in meat and dairy appears to be unfounded. A

2002 Harvard study "found no significant association between intake of meat or dairy products and risk of breast cancer."[8] In fact, a large study conducted in Norway showed that higher cholesterol levels appear to protect against breast cancer.[9] In terms of heart disease, there is no greater risk at cholesterol levels of 300 than at 180.[10] But some research indicates that the "all-cause" death rate is higher in individuals with cholesterol levels lower than 180.[11] This appears to be particularly true for the elderly who show declining physical function and increased frailty when their cholesterol levels drop.[12]

GUILT BY ASSOCIATION

So what is all this business about cholesterol clogging the arteries? Cholesterol is just one part of the plaque that narrows the arteries feeding the heart. Actually, it is more like an innocent bystander in this process. Here's a description of how it appears to work.

To provide its vital functions, cholesterol is transported in the blood by a complex molecule, a lipoprotein. The two major types of lipoproteins are high density (HDL) and low density (LDL). The HDL carries less cholesterol than the LDL and acts like a scavenger. It picks up excess cholesterol and, with the help of plenty of fiber and lecithin in the diet, sends it back to the liver for processing and then excretion.

It is the larger population of cholesterol carriers (the LDL) that attracts the attention of free radicals—you know, those nasty cell-damaging particles that attempt to oxidize the cholesterol and fat held by the LDL. The HDL scavengers, on the other hand, seem to travel along unnoticed and undamaged by the free radicals. This is why it is better to have a higher concentration of this so-called "good cholesterol" in relation to the amounts of LDL—so that there is less LDL around to be oxidized.

Now, once the cholesterol is oxidized, it damages the artery wall, adding to other injuries created by free radicals, or by factors related to pollution, cigarette smoke, stress, and rancid or hydrogenated oils. The immune system tries to repair the damage, creating a patch of foam that accumulates more cholesterol, calcium, platelets, and other debris. This in turn forms a plaque that gets larger and brittle over the years, and then finally—you know the rest—blood flow to the heart is restricted and death can result.

If cholesterol could talk, it might ask, "What did I do wrong?" In this instance, it's a case of guilt by association. Cholesterol just happened to be in the wrong place at the wrong time. Unless the cholesterol becomes oxidized, it creates no harm. Therefore, a great deal of emphasis has been placed on finding ways to prevent LDL cholesterol from becoming oxidized in the bloodstream. Popping more antioxidant supplements is one suggested antidote. Replacing saturated fat with polyunsaturated oils is often recommended so that there is less LDL in the bloodstream. Making dietary changes to increase the ratio of HDL to LDL has gotten a lot of press. But all these suggestions are missing the point. They are leading us astray because the above description of cholesterol's role in cardiovascular disease is not adequate.

A CLEARER PICTURE

A number of our top fat and cholesterol researchers, including Mary Enig, Ph.D., and Uffe Ravnskov, M.D., Ph.D., found too many discrepancies in the widely held view that high levels of cholesterol, particularly LDL, are responsible for heart disease. They note that not only in the United States, but throughout the world, the incidence of heart disease has risen while consumption of animal fat (and cholesterol) has fallen. But, in Switzerland after World War II, heart disease declined as animal fat consumption rose.[13]

Besides the Eskimos with their huge intake of fat and low rates of heart disease, there are tribes in Kenya like the Masai who eat primarily milk, meat, and blood. Sometimes one-half pound of butterfat and several pounds of meat are consumed each day, yet they have no heart disease to speak of and have much lower cholesterol levels than Americans.

Comparing levels of blood cholesterol to rates of heart disease is baffling as well. From the famous Framingham study we find that almost half of those who had heart attacks had low cholesterol. Also from Framingham, after 30 years of study, those whose cholesterol had decreased by itself were at greater risk of dying: "For each 1% m/dl drop of cholesterol there was an 11% increase in coronary and total mortality."[14] We don't often hear this statistic when the subject of Framingham comes up. Usually we hear only the misinterpretations of the Framingham study. We hear only that high cholesterol equals heart disease, although this relationship appeared to exist, not in women, but only in men under the age of 47. For men in Canada, however, there was no relationship shown between high cholesterol and heart disease.[15] What's going on here? When we see that, in France, old women with high levels of cholesterol live the longest,[16] it becomes clear we need a new cholesterol model.

What is being offered as a more accurate way to look at all these apparent discrepancies involves viewing cholesterol not as an innocent bystander and not as an active participant in the heart-disease process. Enig, Ravnskov, and others are telling us that heart disease has multifactoral causes, and that high cholesterol is simply a marker for these other causes. In other words, cholesterol is to be looked at for what it truly is—an essential substance of all cells that promotes membrane and tissue health and that fights against attacks initiated by such things as insulin dysfunction, vitamin and mineral deficiencies, smoking, obesity, stress, depression, and environmental toxins. In short, cholesterol is a healer.

There is no such thing as "bad" cholesterol, unless it is oxidized. Levels of LDL rise specifically to combat assaults on the body, including the cardiovascular system. *Rising cholesterol levels indicate that there is some other problem going on.* Rising cholesterol levels represent something good in the sense that the body is trying to heal itself—like having a fever. The fever is useful in combating viral invaders, and it is counterproductive in most cases to attempt to bring it down. To extend the analogy, if the fever gets out of hand, it must be dealt with. Similarly, those with the genetic problem called "familial hypercholesterolemia" must have their condition treated as well. Their extremely high levels of cholesterol—sometimes up to 1000—indicate that the cholesterol is staying in the bloodstream and is not getting into the tissue where it can be of service. A fever, like most instances of "high" cholesterol, is simply a marker and a healer— an indication that there is some other root cause for symptoms of illness.

THE VALUE OF CHOLESTEROL

When women reach menopause, their LDL levels rise dramatically and they are thought to have a greater risk of heart disease. This greater risk is not likely due to rising cholesterol levels but rather to factors commonly associated with menopause—like hypothyroidism—or to a lack of sleep, which has just recently been identified as an additional risk factor for heart disease. These problems can be compounded by obesity, a sense of social isolation, hypertension, smoking, a sedentary lifestyle, or chronic inflammation. Remember, high cholesterol is a marker for some other event. In older women, especially, higher cholesterol levels are protective.[17] How can this be? Since cholesterol is needed to create progesterone and estrogen, and since these hormones drop off at menopause, it appears that cholesterol is coming to the rescue. The additional cholesterol may be trying its best to create more of these hormones to replace what menopause has taken away. Does it make sense to put menopausal women on cholesterol-lowering drugs to reduce that which is trying to restore hormonal equilibrium?

When under attack, cholesterol levels rise because they need to rise. If arteries are damaged, cholesterol goes to the rescue to repair the injury. Because cholesterol is a part of the plaque in the arteries at the site of the injury, it gets a bad reputation—as does saturated fat. But it needed to be there. When artery clogs are examined we find that about 26 percent of the total fats in the clogs are saturated. The rest is unsaturated, more than half of which is polyunsaturated.[18] The public has been brainwashed into thinking that our arteries clog solely with cholesterol and saturated fat. Not so. Why then hasn't polyunsaturated fat been more positively linked to heart disease? Well, it has—by clear-thinking researchers, but the general public hasn't heard about it. Dr. Bernhard Hennig from the University of Kentucky, while speaking at the American College of Nutrition's 1993 annual conference, claimed that polyunsaturated fats are culprits in the cardiovascular disease process, and he recommended limiting their intake.[19] But this is not what we are usually told. We are more often advised to increase their intake, or at least use them in place of saturated fats. Bad advice.

We are constantly told to lower our fat intake. More bad advice—unless we are talking about the unhealthy *trans* fats or excessive polyunsaturated fats. To illustrate this point, a study from 1998 had subjects reduce their total fat intake to 21 percent of their calories, compared to a control group that continued to consume 41 percent of their calories from fat. In terms of total cholesterol, there was no difference between the two groups. In the lower fat group, however, beneficial HDL declined. Since HDL whisks away unneeded cholesterol, it appears that the lower fat group needed higher levels of cholesterol in the system, which is delivered by the so-called "bad LDL." In other words, the low-fat diet appeared to be showing signs that something was wrong, as evidenced by the lower amounts of HDL. Researchers conducting the study found through testing that those who switched to this lower fat diet showed a significant increase in anger and hostility.[20] Both of those, of course, are risk factors for heart disease, both a result of a diet lower in fat.

We often see studies indicating that formerly healthy groups of people from abroad develop heart disease and other ailments after moving to the United States and eating like the typical American (lots of fat and cholesterol, we are told). According to British physician Dr. Michael Marmot, it's not that simple. He found that among Japanese immigrants, if they maintained their cultural traditions, they were protected against heart attacks even though their diets changed and cholesterol levels increased. The Japanese society puts great emphasis on group support and social stability. Losing a sense of togetherness appears to be a risk factor for heart disease. Dr. Marmot found that those immigrants who maintained the traditional Japanese diet but became accustomed to the American way of life (cowboy individualism, etc.) had coronary heart disease twice as often as those who kept their Japanese traditions but adopted the typical high-fat American diet.[21]

SOME BAD FATS

Unrefined polyunsaturated oils in small amounts can help provide us with some of the essential omega-6 fatty acids our bodies require. A better source for these essential fats would be vegetables, fruits, nuts, seeds, and grains. The public, however, is consuming way too many polyunsaturated oils like corn, safflower, sunflower, cottonseed, and soy. Too many of these fats can upset the balance they must keep with the omega-3 fatty acids, contributing to a number of problems including immune system dysfunction; damage to the liver, reproductive organs, and lungs; digestive disorders; depressed learning ability; impaired growth; and weight gain.[22]

Polyunsaturated oils are easily oxidized, making them a source of free radicals, which injure the arteries and create a situation that cholesterol tries to remedy. Researcher Sally Fallon asks, "Is it any wonder that tests and studies have repeatedly shown a high correlation between cancer and heart disease with the consumption of polyunsaturates?"[23] Not only does cholesterol attempt to repair the lesions created by free-radical damage, it may be helping to prevent such damage in the first place by acting as a potent antioxidant.[24–26]

Companies that sell polyunsaturated oils have been successful with their marketing campaigns to get the public off of butter and onto margarine. Evidence continues to mount, however, which shows the toxic effects of the *trans* fats contained in margarine. Many people now wisely refuse to buy this dangerous food. But many, it appears, are still misled by the marketing ploy: "Polyunsaturated oils are good for you because they lower cholesterol levels." But how do they accomplish this? According to some researchers, a high intake of polyunsaturates weakens cellular membranes. When this occurs cholesterol comes to the rescue once again. Additional cholesterol enters the cell membrane in order to stabilize and restore proper cellular function. In the process, cholesterol is drawn from the bloodstream, thereby lowering serum levels temporarily.[27] This is hailed by marketers as a "success" for their oils, which "reduced cholesterol." In fact, it appears that cholesterol is simply trying to repair the damage done by high levels of polyunsaturated oils. These fats were not common many decades ago when heart disease and certain other chronic diseases were rare.

Research has given us a new way to view cholesterol's relation to disease—one that makes sense, and one that allows us to eat more like our ancestors did, with little regard to the saturated fat or cholesterol content of whole, unprocessed foods. Saturated fat—purported to be very bad for us—is, in fact, extremely important in maintaining the health of the cell membrane, which is comprised of at least 50 percent saturated fatty acids. Saturated fats are also needed for the proper utilization of the essential fatty acids, like the omega-3s,[28] the consumption of which has been shown to reduce the risk of heart attacks.

Cholesterol plays the role of healer. If the task is too big for the role cholesterol attempts to play, and if a person succumbs to heart disease, we wrongly blame the cholesterol instead of focusing on the other factors related to developing this disease. Saturated fat and cholesterol should not be feared.

FRAMINGHAM REVISITED

The Framingham study began in 1948 and is the study most frequently cited in an attempt to link high-fat diets and high cholesterol levels to heart disease. Forty years later, however, the director of the study admitted:

> In Framingham, Mass., the more saturated fat one ate, the more cholesterol one ate, the more calories one ate, the lower the person's serum cholesterol . . . we found that the people who ate the most cholesterol, ate the most saturated fat, ate the most calories, weighed the least and were the most physically active.[29]

WHAT CAN WE DO?

Besides eating whole, nutrient-dense foods, and avoiding excess polyunsaturated and *trans* fats, what other dietary considerations are of value? If the body's cells are happy and healthy with the amount of cholesterol they have taken in, then levels of HDL should rise; the HDL sweeps away cholesterol that is no longer required for repair. Since higher levels of HDL appear to be a marker for good health, researchers have focused on the HDL to LDL ratio—the higher the better. One way to achieve a better ratio is through exercise and by maintaining proper weight. Very fit athletes are known to have high HDL readings. Even moderate exercise like walking creates healthy changes in the body which, in turn, appear to create a demand for fewer of the dense LDL cholesterol particles.[30]

Sugar in the diet is a problem for the heart. Yes, sugar. Even the "natural" fructose found in many soft drinks and "healthy" snack foods can contribute to higher levels of LDL and reduced HDL.[31,32] A diet higher in the essential omega-3 fatty acids (fish, flax, walnuts) helps maintain healthy cholesterol ratios—and, of course, monounsaturated fats like olive oil, which appear to inhibit the oxidation of LDL cholesterol. This sounds a little like the Mediterranean diet.

And speaking of sunny climates, don't forget to get adequate sunlight. Sunlight is vital to countless biological functions. Without sufficient sunlight our bodies are unable to produce vitamin D, which inhibits the growth of cancer cells[33,34] and plays a vital role in maintaining strong bones. Certainly, care must be taken not to get overexposed or sunburned. But some exposure to natural sunlight, perhaps as little as fifteen minutes every other day, is necessary for the body's production of vitamin D.

What does this have to do with cholesterol? Cholesterol is needed to synthesize sunlight into vitamin D. If the body gets inadequate sunlight, cholesterol levels rise. This appears to be a signal that the body is producing more cholesterol in order to synthesize as much of this essential vitamin as it can from low levels of light. Plenty of sunlight then, normalizes cholesterol levels.[35] Once again it is cholesterol's role to protect health rather than to destroy it.

Another strategy to protect the heart is, of course, a diet high in antioxidants. Abundant amounts of fruits and vegetables—and red wine if you're so inclined—will help to prevent oxidative damage to the arteries and also help to keep the cholesterol and fats carried by the LDL from becoming oxidized. A diet high in the vitamin-E complex, for example, provides antioxidants that serve much like a bodyguard. It hitches a ride in the LDL particles in order to protect the cholesterol and fat passengers that are subject to attack by free radicals. For those of you not in love with vegetables (shame on you) supplementing with vitamins C and E, as well as with selenium and CoQ10, would probably be a good idea.

Additionally, avoid cholesterol that has already been oxidized outside the body: dried or powdered milk and eggs. Also on the "to avoid" list are the processed meats. Forget the salami and pepperoni on the pizza. These are the kinds of meats that have been linked to higher rates of cancer. Fresh sources of cholesterol-rich foods are fine. Remember, it's the processed, oxidized, chemical-laden, cholesterol-rich foods that are a problem.

Maintaining a healthy cardiovascular system also appears to involve keeping levels of homocysteine low. This toxic amino acid, created inside the body, was identified as a culprit in artery damage in 1969 by Dr. Kilmer McCully, but his research was either overlooked or ridiculed by mainstream medicine, which could not see past the standard cholesterol theory of heart disease. Now it appears that high levels of homocysteine can contribute not only to heart disease but to osteoporosis as well.[36–39] There even appears to be a link between elevated levels of homocysteine and Alzheimer's disease.[40] In most cases, this substance can be kept in check with a diet supplying plenty of vitamins B_6 (potatoes, bananas, liver, turkey, lentils, wheat bran, cabbage, milk, eggs, cantaloupe) and B_{12}

(eggs, dairy, beef, fish, poultry), folic acid (leafy greens, beans, citrus, beets, meat, carrots, whole wheat) and choline (some of the best sources for choline are egg yolks, lecithin, and fish).

Low-fat, high-carbohydrate diets—particularly those which include large amounts of refined carbohydrates—are also implicated in causing heart disease. The high-carb diets pushed on the public for so many years by numerous health authorities tend to create insulin resistance, whereas a high-fat diet does not.[41] As a result of all the carbs, the body's increased production of insulin not only puts a strain on the pancreas—with diabetic implications—but the excess insulin appears to generate greater levels of heart-damaging homocysteine.[42]

One of the very best ways to maintain cardiovascular health seems to be the easiest: drink plenty of pure water. When cells are healthy and hydrated, cholesterol levels begin to normalize. A recent study of over 20,000 subjects compared those who drank five or more glasses of water a day to those who drank two or less. Fatal heart attacks were cut in half in the group drinking more water. These results represent a better response than from any other regimen or treatment designed to protect the heart. According to the principal investigator, cardiologist Gary Fraser of Loma Linda University, drinking water may be "the cheapest and simplest method of preventing coronary heart disease that could be imagined."[43]

SATURATED FAT

Is there still a concern about saturated fat? Doesn't this fat raise cholesterol levels? Yes, it can. But so what? If cholesterol levels are raised by saturated fat, it is cholesterol created in the body, unoxidized and therefore harmless, or even helpful, in the context of a healthy diet. What is not commonly known is that saturated fat can lower serum cholesterol levels as well. According to lipids researcher Dr. Enig, most fats can either raise or lower cholesterol levels. It depends on whether your levels are low or high to begin with.[44] Saturated fats attempt to normalize cholesterol levels.

With our new cholesterol model, we should now know that high levels in the bloodstream are not the cause of heart disease. Remember, about half of all those having heart attacks have cholesterol readings that are normal or below normal. Furthermore, when saturated fat does raise total cholesterol levels, it has been shown to raise the good HDL in the process.[45,46] In addition to that, and as we have seen from the Framingham study, consumption of saturated fat, a substance absolutely essential to cellular health, lowers a number of markers used by physicians to determine the risk of coronary heart disease.[47]

Excess saturated fat, however, can be a problem due to its tendency to make platelets sticky, causing them to aggregate. This could be trouble for the cardiovascular system if the high amounts of saturated fat are not kept in check by limiting sugar and by increasing fiber.[48] An adequate intake of vitamin C and the essential fats like the omega-3s from fish and flax can also help the general population counteract the effects of excess saturated fat.[49] Another reason why the high saturated fat diet of the Eskimos is not a threat to their cardiovascular systems: they consume plenty of fish oil.

It appears that saturated fat, like cholesterol, isn't the culprit it has been made out to be after all. A recent study of 2000 subjects on a low saturated fat diet for two years showed no reduction in the recurrence of colon tumor precursors.[50] Another 6-year study of 40,000 middle-aged American men showed no link between saturated fat and heart disease.[51] In animal studies as well, saturated fat helped to prevent strokes, not cause them. To say that saturated fat causes heart disease is, as numerous researchers are beginning to point out to us: "Wrong." Even so, the apostles of the low-fat religion are reluctant to loosen their grip on the American diet.

THE EVIL FAT

Fortunately, we frequently see the phrase "good fats and bad fats." If there are some fats that can raise beneficial HDL levels, there are certainly some that can lower these good levels, most notably *trans* fatty acids contained in partially hydrogenated vegetable oils. And these are very bad fats indeed—real killers. But that's not what we were told for so many years. We were told that the hydrogenated oils in margarine would be just the thing to save us from that nasty butter.

Trans fats, however, have been implicated in higher risks of developing both heart disease and cancer. The list of problems associated with the consumption of *trans* fats, unfortunately, is not a short one: heart disease, obesity (by increasing the size of the fat cells), diabetes, low birth weight, allergies, asthma, and immune dysfunction.[52–56] *Trans* fats—created by the deoderization process designed to mask vegetable oil rancidity or through the hydrogenation process to make the oil firm—are found today in countless baked and processed foods. They were identified as unhealthy as far back as 1958. This information was squelched, and a campaign was begun to denigrate the meat and dairy industries in order to promote the sale of vegetable oils.[57]

BEING MISLED

The vegetable oil industry was even clever enough to smear another of its competitors—tropical oils—because the saturated fat in coconut oil, for example, could be linked to that in animal fat and, by extension, to heart disease. Tropical oils have become more vilified even than butter and eggs. Most of us have bought into this deception even though populations consuming high amounts of coconut oil have low rates of heart disease. There are many health-promoting aspects of coconut oil, including its ability to act as an antimicrobial agent. It appears to boost the immune system, and it does not clog the arteries, as we have been led to believe.[58,59]

The Center for Science in the Public Interest (CSPI)—self-described as "a nonprofit public interest organization that advocates improved health and nutrition policies"—for years refused to acknowledge the dangers of *trans* fatty acids. They focused heavily on the supposed dangers of diets high in cholesterol and saturated fat (including coconut oil). Therefore, they even recommended using margarine with its *trans* fats over butter: ". . . Margarine is better for your heart."[60] However, as the research pointing to the dangers of these killer *trans* fats began to mount, CSPI began to change its tune, but not nearly enough. They began to understand some of the problems associated with diets high in these artificial fats, but instead of singling them out, they simply tried to equate them to saturated fats. These two fats act in much different ways in the body. Clean sources of saturated fats can be health-promoting. *Trans* fats do not belong in the diet. A recent report from a panel of experts at the National Academy of Science's Institute of Medicine concluded that the safe amount of *trans* fat in our food is "zero."[61] The typical daily American diet filled with processed foods can contain a staggering 30 grams or more of *trans* fats—which also have been shown to reduce blood-vessel function by 30 percent.[62]

In 1990, the *trans*-fat issue was still not an important one for the folks at CSPI, despite the fact that for decades enlightened researchers had tried to warn government agencies about this danger in our foods. CSPI simply tried to downplay research indicting *trans* fats as a culprit in heart disease by giving us their bottom line: "Trans-shmans"—just eat less fat.[63] Even today, although CSPI calls for labeling the *trans*-fat content in foods, they wish it lumped in with, and not distinguished from, the "dangerous" saturated fats.

It makes you wonder why this self-proclaimed protector of the American diet has not insisted, at the very least, on separate labeling requirements for *trans* fats. A truly enlightened public interest group would call for a complete ban on their use based on the science we have today. Perhaps CSPI is trying to cover themselves for past decisions that may have led to greater widespread use of these dangerous fats, which have been shown to reduce levels of the "good" cholesterol.

CSPI played an active role in two misguided campaigns to remove saturated fats from the American diet and replace them with *trans*-fat-filled hydrogenated vegetable oils.

POPCORN CONTROVERSY

Do you remember the brouhaha over theater popcorn? CSPI was aghast at the amount of saturated fat (coconut oil) in popcorn that was being consumed by the public. Their outcry led theater owners to replace health-promoting coconut oil in popcorn machines with partially hydrogenated vegetable oil, replete with *trans* fats and other artificial substances.

FRENCH FRY WAR

The other campaign involved taking on McDonald's. CSPI no longer wanted French fries cooked in beef tallow, a substance that has been used for centuries as a safe and stable cooking fat. Too much saturated fat, they said. McDonald's and others eventually caved in to the pressure, and so we now have what is perhaps one of the most dangerous foods available—potatoes dripping in toxic, *trans*-fat-soaked vegetable oils.

CSPI had acknowledged the following: "Until the early 1900s, if you wanted a solid fat for your pie crust, you had to choose between lard, butter, or beef tallow. In 1911, Procter and Gamble changed all that when it introduced Crisco, a shortening made by hydrogenating a liquid oil (cottonseed)."[64] It is a mystery why CSPI couldn't put two and two together and see that it was at this very time in our history that heart disease rates began to climb. Healthy, natural animal fats were replaced with polyunsaturated and hydrogenated oils.

Clinging to the myth that saturated fats are bad has led CSPI to apparently increase the amounts of heart damaging, cancer-causing *trans* fats in the American diet. It is interesting to note that, even though CSPI put pressure on McDonald's and then congratulated them for switching to vegetable shortening for the cooking of their fries, they have now recently congratulated McDonald's for reducing the amount of *trans*-fat-laden oils in their popular product.

CSPI has convinced the public that saturated fats are "artery-clogging oils." However, when artery clogs (atheromas) are examined, none of the fatty acids from coconut oils are found. However, plenty of polyun-saturates are found. Coconut oil is the oil of choice when it comes to cooking with high heat because it is so stable and does not easily de-grade into toxic substances like most oils do. It ranks right up there with olive oil and unheated flax oil as the world's healthiest oil. Thanks to the Center for Science in the Public Interest, the public is now as much afraid of coconut oil as it is of anthrax.

MORE ON THE *TRANS* FATS

These nasty fellows disrupt cellular function and interfere with the use of essential fatty acids in the body. For years the FDA turned a blind eye to these facts, although recently they have begrudgingly decided that food labels will soon have to include *trans* fat in the estimation of total fat content. Why not ban it instead of just warning us? One would think that the edible oil industry has the same clout as the tobacco companies.

Instead, this is a product allowed by government in thousands of foods. This is a product suspected of causing death. Breast cancer rates are directly tied to *trans* fat consumption.[65] It is clearly a product that should be banned. It shows up everywhere. It's difficult to find any cracker without the *trans* fats, which are found in "partially hydrogenated vegetable oil." Aside from its oatmeal, most Quaker Oats Company products, for exam-ple, appear to contain some of this cheap, toxic stuff. Even venerable "Ben and Jerry's," a company which, to its credit, does not use milk con-taminated with Monsanto's bovine growth hormone, has some flavors of ice cream that contain partially hydrogenated oil. They say they would like to get rid of it but can't find a suitable replacement. Have they been frightened away from coconut oil?

Government regulations permit products to be labeled as "all natural" even if they have *trans* fats added to them in the form of partially hydro-genated vegetable oil. But the *trans* fats found in these oils do not behave like the *trans* fats that occur naturally in small amounts in certain animal foods like milk. Natural *trans* fats are converted to beneficial conjugated linoleic acid (see the next chapter) or to energy. To say that the partially hydrogenated oil added to countless food products is "natural" is more than a little deceitful.

FOREIGN FAT

As mentioned earlier, rates of heart disease began to rise in the early part of the century when the population began consuming less animal fat and more vegetable oil, although the total percentage of fat intake remained about the same. Another correlation exists: cancer mortality rates have risen along with the increase in vegetable oil consumption.

Some of the blame for cancer must rest with the free radicals that are created by the heating, deodorizing, and refining of vegetable oils, which are stripped of most of their protective vitamin E in the process. But *trans* fats must surely be the most damaging because they are so pervasive and disrupt so many important body processes. A Harvard University study showed higher intakes of *trans* fats in those who developed heart disease.[66]

A significant risk factor for developing heart disease is high levels of a substance in the blood called lipoprotein(a). This Lp(a) is a "sticky" variant of LDL cholesterol and appears to help form arterial plaques. Saturated fat lowers levels of this damaging substance while consumption of *trans* fat raises the amount of Lp(a) in the blood.[67] Cell membranes simply prefer saturated fat, but through their advertising, promoters of the vegetable oil industry have tried to convince us otherwise. A high consumption of polyunsaturated fats, however, has long been connected to the development of cancer and heart disease.[68,69]

It could be asked, however: Since the hydrogenation process converts oils from the polyunsaturated to the saturated form, wouldn't this be OK? No, this is not the kind of saturated fat the body recognizes and can use. It is foreign and toxic. There are those, like CSPI perhaps, who might insist that there isn't enough research to adopt such a hard line on *trans* fats. We might respond by pointing out that the Dutch government has banned the sale of margarine containing *trans* fats. Why don't we? Are the scientists in the Netherlands inept? Or are the Dutch less influenced by the politics of food and by corporate interests? It seems that for some of the folks at the FDA, dietary health in this country is not a top priority. Besides, it's much more convenient to blame it all on cholesterol.

ANOTHER VOICE IN THE WILDERNESS

One of the many experts trying to expose the myth of cholesterol is Dr. Paul J. Rosch. As an author, editor, President of the American Institute of Stress, Expert Consultant on Stress to the U.S. Centers for Disease Control, former President of the New York State Society of Internal Medicine, etc., etc.—Professor Rosch states:

> The public is so brainwashed, that many people believe that the lower your cholesterol, the healthier you will be or the longer you will live. Nothing could be further from the truth. . . . The cholesterol cartel of drug companies, manufacturers of low-fat foods, blood-testing devices and others with huge vested financial interests have waged a highly successful promotional campaign.

Their power is so great that they have infiltrated medical and governmental regulatory agencies that would normally protect us from such unsubstantiated dogma.[70]

Do you suppose that we can finally start to regard moderate amounts of high-quality saturated fats—and the cholesterol they contain—as health foods? Something to ponder. (Woody Allen would be amused.)

■■ TIPS: ■■

There is clinical evidence that stress reduction helps lower cholesterol levels.

Avoid all foods containing partially hydrogenated oils. Start reading labels! Limit sugar—excessive amounts can raise cholesterol levels.

Start adding healthy omega 3s to the diet from fish, flax, walnuts, and olive oil. For cooking at high heat, use organic coconut, sesame, or rice bran oils.

Drink water! It's the easiest way to protect the heart.

CONJUGATED
LINOLEIC ACID

Propaganda: Red meat and dairy products cause heart problems and obesity.

Reality: Grass-fed cows, buffalo, sheep, and goats produce meat and dairy high in heart healthy, weight-reducing conjugated linoleic acid.

CAN BEEF AND BUTTER KEEP YOU THIN?

Sometimes referred to as "the Charles Darwin of nutrition," Weston A. Price traveled much of the world during the 1930s examining the diets of a wide variety of cultures. Dr. Price, a dentist, found a relationship between traditional diets and good dental health, which typically went hand-in-hand with the overall good health of the groups he studied. He found that traditional diets resulted in people free from the typical degenerative diseases that had begun to plague modern society.

What did those cultures eat that seemed to protect them from heart disease, arthritis, diabetes, obesity, and other diseases? What was the common denominator?

Certainly the lack of processed foods containing sugar and white flour stands out. Only whole foods were consumed. But in those whole foods Price found rich and plentiful sources of fat-soluble nutrients. Fish was often found in abundance in the diets of most of the healthiest cultures examined.

Today we recognize the importance of the essential omega-3 fatty acids that are found in large amounts in fish (as well as in flax, walnuts, and other seeds). Recent studies have shown the consumption of omega-3s to be useful in fighting heart disease and inflammatory conditions. These fatty acids boost the immune system and have been shown to protect against cancer.

But what about those healthy cultures in which fish was not a substantial part of the diet? Instead of fish, they consumed large amounts of cheese, butter, and fresh milk from healthy cows allowed to graze on pasture. Dr. Price recognized the value of the fat-soluble vitamin-D complex found in these foods, but he felt there was some other yet-to-be-identified substance found in cow fat that contributed to the health of the populations consuming it. He called it "activator X."

A "Miracle" Nutrient

Decades later researchers may have discovered the identity of a compo-nent of Price's mysterious and health-promoting activator X by acci-dent. In 1978, researchers at the University of Wisconsin, Madison, were attempting to identify cancer-causing compounds called heterocyclic amines (HCAs) that are created when meat is grilled. What turned up was a substance in the beef they were testing that acted as an anticar-cinogen. It was years later before this substance, conjugated linoleic acid (CLA), was isolated and identified.

Found in significant amounts not only in beef fat, but in lamb, buffalo, and other ruminants, CLA is also contained in whole milk, cheese, and butter. Today, research involving this fascinating nutrient is turning heads. Not only has it been shown to inhibit the growth of human breast cancer cells (not to mention malignant melanoma, colorectal, and lung cancer cells),[1-8] animal studies also indicate it lowers LDL cholesterol, resulting in less atherosclerosis—this stuff appears to be good for the heart.[9,10]

Due to the bashing that red meat and full-fat dairy products have taken over the years, people are consuming much less of these foods than they did fifty years ago. In fact, beef consumption has dropped in half during just the last twenty years, according to the USDA. Have cancer and heart disease decreased as a result of our avoidance of these foods? No. It is estimated that during those last twenty years consumption of CLA from animal fat has dropped dramatically while heart disease rates remain high. Furthermore, the current low consumption levels of CLA in the diet are about one-third of that necessary to offer cancer protec-tion (in animal studies).[11] Interestingly, levels of CLA in today's milk due to changed feeding practices (cows are grain-fed instead of allowed to graze) are about one-third of what they were before the 1960s.[12]

An Antifat Fat

The avoidance of foods containing CLA may be a factor contributing to another current malady—obesity. We are fatter than ever today despite eating low-fat this and low-fat that. It has been established that eating essential fatty acids helps the body metabolize other fats more efficiently, thereby contributing to weight loss. Yes, eating the right fats help you lose weight. Well, it also turns out that CLA, a relative of the essential linoleic acid that can only be obtained from food, inhibits fat cells from getting fatter.[13] Human studies have shown that consuming moderate amounts of CLA for three months without dieting resulted in as much as a 20 percent loss of body fat.[14,15] Apparently, CLA affects fat metabolism by interfering with the activity of a fat-regulating hormone, leptin, and possibly by increasing insulin sensitivity. A recent study involving subjects with type-2 diabetes found that consumption of CLA helped them manage their disease by reducing body weight and by lowering blood sugar levels (fivefold, compared to controls).[16] Not only is there a drop in body fat with consumption of conjugated linoleic acid, but CLA appears also to stimulate the development of muscle tissue. Body-builders have certainly taken note of this fact.

The benefits of CLA seem almost too good to be true. No wonder the groups eating plenty of butter and cheese studied by Weston Price seemed so fit. Perhaps today's "French Paradox" is due not solely to the consumption of red wine, but also of full-fat dairy products.

And just when you thought it couldn't get any better, there is substantive evidence that CLA has antioxidant capabilities.[17] Is this a miracle or what? Are you ready to rush down to the local market and grab up all the beef and cheese you've been longing for all these years? Not so fast.

MEAT AND DAIRY ARE NO LONGER WHAT THEY USED TO BE

Typical supermarket beef and milk are not recommended for anyone. Cattle-raising practices over the years have yielded meat that is contaminated with hormones and antibiotics, as well as pesticide residue from the grains fed to the animals. Today's typical beef contains an unnatural, overabundance of the omega-6 fatty acids. Not only that, animals fed hay and grains have a much lower CLA content. Ruminants have digestive tracts that convert the linoleic acid in food they eat into CLA, and when their food is green grass, the CLA content of the meat, or the milk, is many times higher.[18] Grain-fed beef today is deficient not only in CLA but also in the healthy omega-3 fatty acids.

Therefore, a search for organically raised beef is well worth the effort, particularly if the animals are allowed to graze. A good option would be to look for buffalo meat. Typically, buffalo are not fed hormones, and they eat plenty of grass. And if you are concerned about the carcinogens formed when grilling meat, be informed that in the case of ground beef, the CLA content actually rises as much a five times from this cooking practice.[19] What symmetry! Grilling creates the carcinogenic HCAs and at the same time raises the levels of an anticarcinogen. CLA is very stable and is not affected by heating, canning, or other preparation methods.

By the way, emptying the contents of a vitamin E capsule into ground beef before grilling is a good way to protect against the formation of HCAs, which are greatly inhibited by this antioxidant.[20] It should be noted that university researchers offering this useful tip used powdered vitamin E capsules. Meats should always be cooked at the lowest possible temperatures to minimize the production of harmful substances. It's high time that we resurrect those old crock-pots that have been hiding in the back of our cupboards all these years.

With cuts of meat or fish to be grilled, another large reduction in harmful HCAs can be obtained by marinating the pieces first.[21,22] Some marinades, especially those that are vinegar-based, have reduced HCAs by as much as 99 percent.[23] Barbecue sauce, on the other hand, has been shown to increase levels of dangerous HCAs.[24] Researchers speculate that it may be the high sugar content of such sauces that leads to higher amounts of these carcinogens.

COWS ON DRUGS

Supermarket milk is subject to the same contamination and problems plaguing meat, with a couple of additions. The specific growth hormone used on many dairy herds (rBST) appears to create higher levels of a specific protein that is linked to cancer. This protein generated by the addition of rBST is said to be more unstable than usual and, according to one expert, enhances diabetes in people prone to the disease. In rat studies, rBST entered the intestinal tract and resulted in a weakened immune system. (See the chapter titled "Bovine Growth Hormones.")

The use of this hormone began in 1993 when Monsanto sought approval of its product from the FDA. Informative studies about the dangers of this hormone were either ignored or suppressed, and the FDA apparently said to Monsanto: "Sure, whatever you want."

Scientists in the Canadian government have been more thorough— or at least less swayed by corporate influence. They have rejected the use of this hormone.

Another downside to many commercial brands of milk is the homogenization process it goes through. Homogenization blends the fat globules with the rest of the milk so that the cream does not rise to the top. This milk fat contains an enzyme called xanthine oxidase (XO), which is suspected of being a potent cause of heart disease because of the damage it does to arterial walls.[25] Normally, in unhomogenized milk, this enzyme is not absorbed by humans, but thanks to homogenization, the newly emulsified milk fat releases XO, making it available for absorption into the bloodstream. In countries like the United States where homogenized milk is commonly consumed, heart attack rates are much higher than in those countries where this process is less common.

Unless you cannot digest dairy products or are allergic to the proteins in milk, look for organic milk products, or better yet, raw milk products. The milk consumed by Dr. Price's healthy cultures was raw. Such milk is difficult to obtain today as a result of our fear of bacterial contamination. If raw milk from dairies can be properly monitored to provide pathogen-free raw milk, what a boon this would be to the nutritional well-being of the public. When cows eat grass—as they were designed to, or even hay, the amounts of dangerous *E. coli* are reduced and altered in such a way as to make it difficult to infect the human gastric system.[26] If milk is pasteurized, many protective health-promoting nutrients are destroyed. This might explain the sudden rise in heart disease that occurred within two years after the introduction of high heat pasteurization—perhaps in those who depended on the nutrients in milk.[27] When purchasing organic milk, ask if the cows graze during the spring and summer to assure the highest possible content of CLA. And don't forget cheese. Even plain old cheddar cheese increases levels of CLA in the body.[28,29] Organic cheese—a health food—isn't life great? (No secret to the French.)

A CANCER FIGHTER

Can all this good news about CLA be true? Is it proven? For the last few years researchers have been cautious. They would say that the animal studies were "promising." Or that they were just "preliminary" studies. It is wise to be cautious, but currently there is more cause to celebrate: A recent study from France has shown that, for humans, CLA intake is related to a 74 percent reduced risk of breast cancer and its recurrence.[30] Another more recent study from Finland, where raw milk is available, found a reduced risk of breast cancer in women consuming more dairy foods.[31] And in Norway, 2002 research found that women who consumed more milk had less breast cancer.[32] From the Netherlands, consumption of fermented milk products like yogurt and buttermilk also reduced the risk of breast cancer.[33] Women with breast cancer have lower CLA levels in their blood than those without this disease.[34] It is theorized that CLA becomes a part of the immune system, which identifies whether or not a particular cell is a normal cell or a cancer cell. If there is a lack of CLA, cancer cells are not as easily recognized and are less likely to be killed by the immune system.[35]

It is sad to think that so many women, in particular, have been persuaded by advertising and by politically correct advice into giving up whole milk in favor of less nutritious drinks like skim milk, or worse yet, soy milk. On the other hand, it could be argued, why bother with milk or red meat at all? Why not just gobble up the CLA pills? Yes, they are available now in all the health food stores. Sounds like a good deal—get cancer protection, weight loss, and a healthy heart—all from a bottle, and pretty cheap at that.

FOOD, NOT PILLS

The point that Weston Price and others have emphasized is that true health is a result of a good diet, a diet of whole foods, a diet of traditional foods. To get an excess of a particular nutrient may not be wise. There are even problems associated with too many calcium tablets or vitamin C pills (see pp. 93–99). It is usually best to get the nutrients in the context in which they are found in nature. Fish oil supplements may be an exception because of the difficulty today in obtaining fish from uncontaminated waters.

Although body-builders are swallowing CLA pills by the handful, there is more than idealistic theory advising against this practice. As you will discover, some research seems to indicate that excessive vitamin C can begin to act in an oxidative manner, instead of remaining the antioxidant hero we are used to. With CLA supplements, a similar thing seems to occur. Subjects taking 4.2 grams of CLA a day for three months experienced an increase in lipid peroxidation—meaning an increase in free-radical production—not a good thing.[36] So, again, caution with high doses of supplements is called for. Eating traditional foods grown and raised the old-fashioned way is the best preventative medicine.

■■ TIPS: ■■

Organic meat and dairy from grass-fed animals are higher in CLA and omega 3s.

Add the contents of a vitamin E capsule into ground beef before grilling to counter carcinogens.

FLUORIDATION

Propaganda: Fluoride prevents tooth decay and is a harmless additive found in toothpaste, rinses, and our water supply.

Reality: Fluoride is a cumulative poison, which thirteen countries have banned. Half of what we eat collects in teeth and bones, making them dense but brittle. Among other conditions, fluoride can cause dental fluorosis, which signals systemic fluoride poisoning.

THE POISONING OF AMERICA, PART I

If you now suspect there is too much fluoride in green tea that could contribute to skeletal damage and hypothyroidism, and have decided to drink something else, how about the small amount added to water supplies serving about 60 percent of the population to bring the total fluoride content to about one part per million? Too little to do any harm?

First, fluoride is, as you know, one of the most toxic substances on earth, on par with arsenic and lead. It has no proven biological use inside the human body (teeth included). There is no minimum daily requirement for fluoride. And second, it is a cumulative poison. Only about half of what we consume is excreted. The other half collects in the teeth and bones, making them dense, but brittle. Those little white spots visible on the teeth of about 25 percent of American children are called dental fluorosis, a condition which not only predisposes them to decay,[1] but also provides a sign that systemic fluoride poisoning is taking place. Dental fluorosis appears to serve as a red flag for future bone fractures as well.[2]

Not only are the teeth of children with those spots damaged, but this fluorosis also indicates that their thyroid glands are being negatively impacted. Increasing rates of learning problems and hyperactivity among American children are thought to be traced in part to thyroid problems,[3] which can be linked to intakes of fluoride. Significant amounts of lead, which accompany the fluoride in most artificially fluoridated systems, are also associated with learning and behavioral problems in children.[4] The impact on the thyroid of adults from fluoride consumption is significant as well. Joint pains, increased cholesterol levels, depression, fatigue, and weight gain are some of the symptoms of a hypothyroid condition. These are the same symptoms of fluoride poisoning, and have occurred from drinking water containing the usual one part per million. This has led to the banning of fluoride in Holland.[5]

BRAIN AND HORMONE PROBLEMS

It has recently been discovered that fluoride also accumulates in the pineal gland, thereby lowering the production of the important regulatory hormone, melatonin.[6] A deficit of melatonin can result in the onset of early sexual maturation in children. In addition, lowered amounts of melatonin increase the risk for breast cancer in women.[7] Hypothyroidism also predisposes women to breast cancer. The prevalence of fluoride in this country—with its impact on the thyroid gland—must certainly be considered one of the contributory factors in our obesity epidemic. Incidentally, the thyroid drug, Synthroid™, was the fourth most-prescribed drug in the United States in the year 2000.

The neurotoxic nature of fluoride is also linked to motor dysfunction, IQ deficits, and learning disabilities.[8] To compensate for poisoning our children, the medical establishment seems to have no other solution than to drug our children with Ritalin. Though hyperactivity is certainly multifactoral, it is on the rise, and it is interesting to note that European countries that have banned fluoridation (thirteen of them—now that Switzerland has recently joined the list) appear to have lower rates of hyperactivity among their children. Or are they simply less apt to medicate their children than we are? Nevertheless, in the year 2000, a group of Boston physicians concluded: "Studies in animals and human populations suggest that fluoride exposure, at levels that are experienced by a significant proportion of the population whose drinking water is fluoridated, may have adverse impacts on the developing brain."[9]

Officials in government health agencies, however, like former Surgeon General C. Everett Koop, believe that the early warning sign of fluoride poisoning—dental fluorosis—is just a "cosmetic problem." This is nonsense. Those spots represent areas of the tooth that have been damaged. If Mr. Koop and the other bureaucrats at the EPA had been honest in claiming that fluorosis was more than cosmetic in nature, they would have been forced by law to act on getting fluoride out of the environment—something they did not want to do. In the long term, people with fluoride-damaged teeth wind up with more spots, more decay, and fewer teeth. Decay rates in fluoridated areas are about the same as in unfluoridated cities, yet dentists historically earn more money in communities that artificially fluoridate their water.[10] Recently, in California, dental costs have fallen in nonfluoridated communities but continued to rise in fluoridated ones.[11] Rising rates of dental fluorosis are suspected as a culprit in increased costs.

Scientists at the EPA have long known about fluoride's dangers and have attempted to bring about some reductions in the amount the public is exposed to. Some have openly spoken about the health problems associated with fluoridated water. Chief Toxicologist, Dr. William Marcus, was even fired from the EPA for voicing his concerns. Scientists there have personally seen how chronic fatigue and fibromyalgia symptoms are associated with consuming water "optimally" fluoridated at one part per million. They have called for a national moratorium on water fluoridation.

Their supervisors, however, are not listening. Currently, there is a battle being waged at the EPA. The union of scientists is attempting to force the EPA leadership to set a policy in which scientific integrity is restored—to set in place rules allowing scientists to conduct research without their findings being ignored or changed to suit the whim of various political interests. They no longer want to experience what one employee was told recently by an EPA boss: "It's your job to support me, even if I say 2 + 2 = 7."[12]

AN "OFFICIAL" CONTAMINANT

The EPA officially lists fluoride as a water contaminant, yet permits its addition to water. Doesn't that sound odd? Public water supplies may have no more than four parts per million. This figure was set because long-term ingestion of this much typically results in crippling skeletal effects. So then one part per million is safe? No amount is safe because it accumulates in the body. In addition, because there is so much fluoride in the environment from all sources (the food chain, pollution, pesticides), the estimated average daily intake of six to seven milligrams (6–7 ppm)[13] almost guarantees future skeletal problems. Consumption of fluoride has recently been positively linked to increased rates of osteoarthritis.[14] This substance damages joints as well as kills bone cells.[15] It is estimated that there are already millions of elderly people suffering from arthriticlike symptoms of some degree due to decades of drinking fluoridated water and beverages made with such water, and the number is certain to rise.

The toxic effects of fluoridated water are amplified by the type of fluoride added. Ninety percent of the fluoride added to our water comes from extremely toxic waste (silicofluorides). Aluminum and fertilizer factories are heavy polluters. They attempt to recover many of the contaminants that would otherwise escape through their smokestacks with devices called scrubbers. The highly toxic junk collected from the scrubbers would cost corporations about $8000 a truckload to properly dispose of (almost $600 million per year).[16] Besides fluoride, this poisonous soup contains varying amounts of lead, cadmium, mercury, radium, arsenic, and other contaminants. So instead of paying to dispose of this material in a toxic dump site, the aluminum and fertilizer indutries actually get paid for it. Cities throughout the country buy this witches' brew, which contains less than 20 percent total fluoride, add it to their water supplies, and claim they are performing a public service—it is actually a corporate service. Industry is quite happy about this arrangement because of the millions of dollars it saves annually.

This form of fluoride (silicofluorides) has never undergone any independent, scientifically valid, double-blind testing to see if it is safe. The FDA calls it an "unapproved drug." If it is unapproved, how can they allow it in our water? How can they allow the entire country to be contaminated with it? Its use in canned foods and drinks and in dental products reaches even those who drink only bottled water. Could corporate profits have something to do with the reason why we haven't joined most of the world in refusing to add this substance to our drinking water?

FRAUDULENT SCIENCE

Perhaps, a more interesting question is: How did we get tricked into poisoning ourselves in the first place? There must have been some evidence that fluoride would help to prevent tooth decay. The initial evidence came in 1939 from a dentist working with the U.S. Public Health Service, H. Trendley Dean. He looked at the incidence of tooth decay in 345 Texas communities. He found that communities with natural fluoride levels of one part per million in their water had fewer cavities (although 10 percent of them had white spots—mild dental fluorosis described as "beautiful white teeth.")

Dr. Dean used a strategy called "selective use of data." This means he used only the data that supported his point of view. He used data from only 21 communities to prove that fluoride at 1 ppm reduced cavities. He completely disregarded data collected from 272 other localities that showed almost no correlation between fluoride and tooth decay.[17] But the stage was set, and the fluoride juggernaut was ready to roll. It needed just one big push. And it got that push from the Manhattan Project, the military program that developed the atomic bomb. This startling information was recently uncovered by investigative reporters Joel Griffiths and Chris Bryson while working for the *Christian Science Monitor*, which subsequently refused to print their discoveries.[18]

Fluoride was crucial to the bomb makers. It was needed to help process uranium; tons of it were needed. During the mid-1940s the DuPont Corporation supplied the military's Manhattan Project with the fluoride it required. There was a big problem, however. The area in New Jersey surrounding the DuPont plant was being contaminated by toxic fluoride emissions. People became ill, cattle and horses were crippled, and crops were either contaminated or completely wiped out. Naturally, the farmers in the area were angry and were ready to sue DuPont and the military, both of whom were keeping silent concerning how much fluoride was being released into the environment.

In preparation for the impending court battle—and to head off any bad publicity that might negatively impact the fluoride/bomb production—the Manhattan Project authorized the military to conduct its own fluoride studies. Not only did they want information that would help diffuse the farmers' anger, they also needed to know to what extent the chemical workers were being harmed from fluoride exposure.

MORE FRAUD

Some of the lab studies were performed at Strong Memorial Hospital, the same facility that injected toxic, radioactive plutonium into unsuspecting human guinea pigs. Research from that time showed that fluoride had a negative impact on the central nervous system. This corroborates recent research showing the same thing—to the extent that the IQs of children in fluoridated areas are lower than normal.[19,20] Other information and studies from the 1940s are apparently still "classified" or have "disappeared."

Still needing "facts" that would calm public fears about fluoride's dangers, the work of Dr. Dean was seized upon to launch a 10-year study of the benefits that fluoridated water would have for dental health. With this fluoridation trial in Newburgh, New York, the military could further study the effects of fluoride as well as initiate a public relations campaign that would eventually enable them to declare that fluoride was safe. Much like the plutonium studies, Newburgh's citizens were being used as test subjects.

The aluminum industry was also eager to get the fluoride bandwagon rolling. They had been marketing their fluoride waste as a rat poison and insecticide and were looking for a larger market. With the influence and urging of Dr. Dean's mentor, Andrew Mellon of the U.S. Public Health Service, who was also the founder and a major stockholder of Alcoa Aluminum, tests were planned to prove to the public that fluoride in water would reduce the incidence of cavities.

Therefore, a 10-year trial began in Michigan in 1945. To make the research "scientifically valid," two cities would be compared. Grand Rapids would be fluoridated and Muskegon would not. About halfway through the study, however, it was discovered that tooth decay rates in Grand Rapids had indeed fallen. But decay rates also fell in unfluoridated Muskegon at about the same rate. With pressure from the bomb producers, and at the urging of public health agencies, Muskegon was dropped from the study; the data from that city was never published.

HEALTH ORGANIZATIONS CLIMB ON BOARD

Despite the fact that the original 10-year study was not completed as planned, Muskegon was hastily fluoridated, and despite the fact that there was no clear evidence that fluoride was either safe or effective, water fluoridation was then declared a triumph for public health. All this occurred not long after the *Journal of the American Dental Association* had warned in an editorial in 1944 that " . . . the potentialities for harm (from fluoridation) far outweigh those for the good." According to Dr. Charles Gordon Heyd, past president of the American Medical Association: "I am appalled at the prospect of using water as a vehicle for drugs. Fluoride is a corrosive poison that will produce serious effects on a long-range basis. Any attempt to use water this way is deplorable." No matter. Despite their former opposition, both the ADA and the AMA joined the fluoride bandwagon based on this fraudulent research.

In 1955, only five years after the widespread acceptance and practice of water fluoridation, H. Trendley Dean (the "father of fluoridation") admitted under oath in a court case challenging fluoridation that his conclusions—the ones upon which the efficacy of fluoridation are based— were wrong.[21] Again, no matter. Decades later we are still adding this toxin to our water.

The public continues to be misled. Many are confused. A few facts about the dangers of fluoride leak out here and there, but when the public seeks reassurance from public health officials or from their own dentists, they are told not to worry—that countless studies have proven fluoride to be safe and effective. Sadly, as a rule, dentists know little about the facts. They merely parrot the propaganda fed to them by the American Dental Association.

The problem is compounded when the public listens to health "authorities" they trust—such dispensers of health wisdom like talk radio's Dr. Dean Edell, who tells his followers that fluoride is one of our "best preventative efforts,"[22] or alternative medicine guru Andrew Weil, who recommends fluoride supplements for pregnant women,[23] even though this toxin passes right through the placenta to the brain of the unborn. Fluoride tablets, drops, and chewing gum have all been banned recently in Belgium—the first nation to do so—because it was felt the poisonous nature of this substance posed a great risk to children's health. Water fluoridation had already been banned there.

When fluoride's safety is questioned, people with legitimate concerns are often treated with disdain. They are told that fluoride in "optimal" amounts is safe—the studies say so. The promoters and defenders of this toxin need to be asked: "What studies?" When old and/or faulty research (by today's standards) is tossed out, including that from other countries, like the recent *York Review* (of fluoridation) in which important data was omitted or misinterpreted, there remain no reliable studies confirming the safety of water fluoridation. None. Zero. There are not even any double-blind studies showing fluoride's effectiveness.[24] There are, however, over 500 peer-reviewed studies showing adverse effects from fluoride.

TELLING IT LIKE IT IS

Thanks to researchers like Canada's Andreas Schuld, the public is becoming more informed. Schuld, a musician and record producer, got involved when his daughter was seriously poisoned. None of the typical household poisons were involved. Andreas needed to find the cause and eventually traced it to grape juice. Yes, grape juice. Grape juice with very high levels of a fluoride-containing pesticide. This launched the establishment of PFPC (Parents of Fluoride Poisoned Children). Andreas Schuld is now one of the world's most knowledgeable people concerning fluoride toxicity. Besides detailing how the thyroid is damaged from the unacceptable amounts of fluoride found in everyday food items from grapes to green tea, he has brought to light some of the following research, keeping in mind that today's estimated average fluoride intake is 6–7 mg per day (6–7 ppm):

- The National Academy of Science in 1977 reported that, for the average individual, a retention of 2 mg per day would result in crippling skeletal fluorosis after 40 years.
- *JAMA*: At the level of 0.4 ppm, renal (kidney) impairment has been shown.
- Half a tube of fluoridated toothpaste can kill a child. (Have you seen the warning on the toothpaste labels?)
- Since there is no regulated dose requirement, children have died in the dentist's chair upon receiving fluoride treatments.
- In 1990 fluoride was found to be an equivocal carcinogen by the National Cancer Institute Toxicology Program. In 1992 further studies by the New Jersey Department of Health confirmed a 6.9-fold increase in bone cancer in young males living in fluoridated areas.[25] (In the lab, male rats are more likely to get cancer from fluoride.)

- There have been five epidemiological studies done since 1990, in three different countries, all showing a higher increase in hip fractures in fluoridated communities. Some studies have indicated an 87 percent higher risk of hip fractures to the elderly in areas where water fluoridation was below 1.5 ppm.
- According to Dr. William Hirzy, vice-president of the union that represents all of the scientists at the EPA (a union calling for a moratorium on water fluoridation): IQ levels were significantly lower in children exposed to fluorides in all age groups listed—5 to 19 points lower! This also explains a recent University of South Florida study connecting fluoride intake during pregnancy to the yearly 1 percent increase in learning disabilities found in children.
- There are several studies linking aluminum with fluoride, showing that aluminum is absorbed more completely in the presence of fluoride. The aluminum in the brains of test animals doubles when accompanied by fluoride, resulting in brain tangles (amyloid deposits). Fluoride is neurotoxic by itself, but becomes many times more toxic when combined with aluminum. This leads to strong speculation that increasing rates of Alzheimer's disease correspond to increasing ingestion of fluoride.[26-28] (It should be noted that most soft drinks and some beers are made with fluoridated water. When consuming these beverages from aluminum cans, the fluoride/aluminum combination is particularly dangerous.)

FURTHER CANCER CONCERNS

With regard to cancer, biochemist John Yiamouyiannis and Dr. Dean Burk, chief Chemist Emeritus of the National Cancer Institute, published a paper in 1975 that detailed an increase in cancer deaths in fluoridated areas. They found that more than 10,000 Americans were dying from cancer each year as a result of the fluoride in their water. According to Dr. Burk, "In point of fact, fluoride causes more human cancer, and causes it faster, than any other chemical."[29]

Using fraudulent tactics, health agencies tried their best to discredit the study. Congressional hearings were held—as well as a court trial in Pennsylvania. In both instances the excess cancer deaths were confirmed. Court Judge John P. Flaherty pointed out that he was "compellingly convinced" of the adverse effects of fluoridation. He ordered a halt to fluoridation as a public health hazard. But the stoppage did not take hold despite the evidence. Our public health agencies wield too much power. It appears that it is our government's intent to take whatever steps are necessary to dispose of this toxic waste through our water supply.

Fortunately, the evidence against fluoride continues to mount. In the year 2000 a research team from Dartmouth College released a study that examined the levels of lead in the blood of over 400,000 children in three different samples. In each case lead levels were higher in those who drank water treated with silicofluorides—the industrial waste added to the water of 140,000,000 Americans.

The effects of lead on the brains of children are devastating, to say the least. In fact, the most recent studies concerning the ability of lead to lower the IQs of children confirm earlier research. In addition, it has now been found that low, "acceptable" levels of lead are more toxic to children than previously thought. Scientists are now advising that there is absolutely no "safe" level of lead exposure. Will we, then, continue to add this toxin to our water along with its fluoride partner?

Like the union of scientists at the EPA, Dartmouth College research team leader Roger D. Master, a Nelson A. Rockefeller Professor of Government Emeritus, called for a moratorium on fluoridating water with these silicofluoride compounds. He added that such substances "have effects like the chemical agents linked to Gulf War Syndrome, chronic fatigue syndrome, and other puzzling conditions that plague millions of Americans."[30]

Will Professor Master's voice be lost along with those of countless other researchers and award-winning scientists, including fourteen Nobel Prize winners, who have spoken the truth about water fluoridation? Will the work and words of Albert Shatz, the codiscoverer of the cure for tuberculosis, be forgotten? Dr. Shatz has called fluoridation the greatest fraud ever perpetuated, and in court testimony concerning the high infant mortality rate of children in Chile following fluoridation of drinking water, Dr. Shatz claimed: "It is my best judgment, reached with a high degree of scientific certainty, that fluoridation is invalid in theory and ineffective in practice as a preventative of dental caries. It is dangerous to the health of consumers."[31] As new research emerges, which substantiates what prominent scientists have proclaimed for decades, a shift in the wind is apparent. We have a faint hope that common sense will prevail.

CAT OUT OF THE BAG

In the July 2000 issue of the *Journal of the American Dental Association*, an article at long last revealed a well-kept secret: Dental Professor J. D. B. Featherstone of the University of California at San Francisco pointed out that the systemic ingestion of fluoride has little effect on the prevention of cavities.[32] The stuff only works when it is applied topically, as with toothpaste, largely because the fluoride in it is such a strong poison: It kills the bacteria on the teeth that lead to decay. Prof. Featherstone, however, is not yet ready to abandon the sinking fluoride ship. He claims that every little bit helps—the assumption being that it would be a good idea to swish the fluoridated tap water around in your mouth frequently in order to get the greatest benefit from fluoride's topical effects. Apparently, we are supposed to accept the fact that industrial waste is being piped into our homes so that we all have access to free mouthwash.

If fluoride then only works topically, why are we still saturating our tissues with it through the water we drink and the water we bathe in? Why are pregnant mothers advised to take fluoride supplements? Why are fluoride drops rubbed on the gums of babies who don't yet have any teeth? Why does much of the public still equate fluoride with mom, baseball, and apple pie? Why do we listen to the majority in the dental community whose ignorance is only partly justified by its good intentions?

ADMITTING A MISTAKE

Hardy Limeback, head of the Department of Preventive Dentistry for the University of Toronto, once belonged to a group of dental professionals who gave talks to promote the benefits of water fluoridation. He was one of Canada's primary promoters of public fluoridation—until he began to take a closer look at the research. He noticed the higher incidence of hip fractures. He noticed the mottled and brittle teeth. Dr. Limeback notes: "Here in Toronto we've been fluoridating for 36 years. Yet Vancouver—which has never fluoridated—has a cavity rate lower than Toronto's." He warns that children under three should never use fluoridated toothpaste. With regard to the water: "Because of the cumulative properties of the toxins, the detrimental effects on human health are catastrophic."

Recently, Dr. Limeback admitted that the truth was a bitter pill to swallow. He apologized to students and faculty at the University of Toronto for unintentionally misleading his colleagues: "For the past 15 years, I had refused to study the toxicology information that is readily available to anyone. Poisoning our children was the furthest thing from my mind."

He added: "Your well-intentioned dentist is simply following 50 years of misinformation from public health and the dental association. Me, too. Unfortunately, we were wrong."[33]

■■ TIP: ■■
Only distillation or reverse osmosis filtration can remove fluoride from tqp water.

ASPARTAME

Propaganda: The American Diabetic Association recommends the use of aspartame to lower blood sugar. Consuming aspartame, as opposed to sugar, can reduce body weight.

Reality: Aspartame is linked to many nervous system disorders, as well as to brain cancer, and can exacerbate some symptoms of diabetes. The American Cancer Society has noted that those who use artificial sweeteners gain more weight than those who don't, and there is evidence that aspartame is addictive.

THE POISONING OF AMERICA, PART II

Betty Martini is an aspartame activist. She created quite a stir in 1995 when a letter she wrote, based on her talks at the World Environmental Conference that year, found its way to the Internet as the "Nancy Markle" letter.[1] It was widely circulated and shocked the world. She clearly laid out the dangers of aspartame consumption and showed how government and corporate interests put profits ahead of public health.

Ms. Martini said, "If you are using aspartame (NutraSweet™, Equal™, Spoonful™, etc.) and you suffer from fibromyalgia symptoms, spasms, shooting pains, numbness in your legs, cramps, vertigo, dizziness, headaches, tinnitus, joint pain, depression, anxiety attacks, slurred speech, or memory loss—you probably have Aspartame Disease!" She pulled no punches. This is quite a shopping list. But is it based on good science? Indeed it is.

She was attacked, however, by some who felt the information belonged to the category of "urban legend" or "urban rumor." One prominent critic said that she left too many unanswered questions. When Ms. Martini answered those questions, her critic refused to put them on his Web site.

Another so-called "exposer of junk science" who tried to discredit her position over the Internet was, in fact, a former lobbyist for the tobacco industry and directed an organization created by Philip Morris to attack the EPA's position on second-hand smoke. He and other shills working for industry front-groups have formed much of Ms. Martini's opposition.

Sadly, many people are misled by those seemingly self-appointed "quackbusters" who hide their affiliation with industry and attempt to discredit those who present facts that contradict widely held beliefs—facts that could hurt corporate profits. Unfortunately, the public is often quick to agree with them because of its unwillingness or inability to accept the possibility that government agencies like the FDA are not protecting us as they should.

WHAT'S IN ASPARTAME?

Betty Martini points out that aspartame contains methanol, or wood alcohol, the very same substance that has blinded or killed so many skid-row alcoholics. This methanol, besides being toxic, is cumulative, converting to formaldehyde, which is a known carcinogen. When found in nature, methanol coexists with ethanol, which acts as a buffer and neutralizes the effects of methanol.[2] In aspartame, there is no such buffer.

The EPA has set a maximum safety limit of methanol consumption at 7.8 mg per day. A one-liter container of "diet" or "sugar-free" soda contains 56 mg. Researchers suggest that the consumption of this poison can trigger or worsen multiple sclerosis, brain tumors, epilepsy, chronic fatigue symptoms, Parkinson's disease, Alzheimer's disease, mental retardation, birth defects, fibromyalgia, diabetes, hyperactivity, and symptoms of lupus.[3-8]

Another ingredient in aspartame is the amino acid phenylalanine, which, in excess, changes brain chemistry. Phenylalanine found in food sources is typically metabolized slowly by the body with no ill effects, unless one has the genetic condition called phenylketonuria (PKU) and cannot metabolize it well at all. Such people must definitely avoid aspartame and foods containing this amino acid. Those not afflicted with PKU, however, can develop high blood levels of phenylalanine by consuming Nutrasweet™—levels that are suspected of lowering serotonin levels and leading to emotional disorders.[9] It breaks down the seizure threshold, causing manic depression and panic attacks. According to neurosurgeon Dr. Russell Blaylock: "The ingredients (in aspartame) stimulate the neurons of the brain to death causing brain damage of varying degrees."[10]

CANCER HYPOTHESIS

What about statistics? Have rates of brain cancer, for example, been tracked? Have they risen since the use of aspartame in food began in 1981, and in soft drinks in 1983? Yes, according to Prof. John Olney and colleagues of Washington University, St. Louis.[11] He noticed that the incidence of brain cancer jumped 10 percent after the introduction of aspartame, most notably between 1984 and 1985. This represents an extra 1500 cases of brain cancer per year, with a sharp increase in the more aggressive type of cancer.[12] Perhaps not coincidentally, it was the development of brain cancer in laboratory animals that held up the approval of aspartame for so many years. Scientists were finding that animals developed brain tumors from aspartame when it broke down into a brain-tumor agent called DKP (diketopiperazine).

Prof. Olney has been criticized for linking aspartame to higher rates of brain cancer. His critics use a study by the National Cancer Institute showing that brain cancer rates actually began to rise in 1973—before aspartame use. Olney points out that, although this may be true, the spike in the rate of brain tumors in 1984 and 1985 indicates that some carcinogen—such as aspartame—had to be introduced suddenly, as opposed to other toxins that enter the environment more gradually.

His critics, including those in the food industry, such as the National Soft Drink Association, have called his ideas "preposterous," claiming, "It is physiologically impossible for aspartame to be a carcinogen—it never enters the bloodstream."[13] Wrong. This kind of blatant misinformation is what keeps the public confused, and the Nutrasweet™ industry in business.

Dr. Joseph Mercola, osteopath and author of numerous articles on Nutrasweet™, claims that about 80 percent of all food complaints to the FDA are for adverse reactions to aspartame, including five reported deaths.[14–16] He notes that in 1991 the National Institutes for Health listed 167 symptoms and reasons to avoid aspartame. Those who fly planes need to avoid aspartame for sure. There have been over 600 calls to the Aspartame Consumer Safety Network reporting symptoms of aspartame poisoning from airplane pilots alone, some of whom reported grand mal seizures while in the cockpit. In 1992 the U.S. Air Force issued an alert about pilots consuming aspartame.[17] The issue of seizures with aspartame consumption is certainly of concern.[18,19]

DIABETICS AND CHILDREN

But doesn't the American Diabetic Association recommend the use of aspartame, despite evidence that it causes blood sugar to go out of control and exacerbate some of the symptoms of diabetes? Don't they recommend it even though, according to Ms. Martini, some diabetics have suffered memory loss, gone into a coma, and died? Yes. Unfortunately the American Diabetic Association and the American Dietetic Association reportedly receive funding from the manufacturer of aspartame.

A diabetes specialist, Dr. H. J. Roberts has pinpointed another problem with aspartame—one of many problems documented in his 1000-page book on the topic. He claims that consuming it at the time of conception can cause birth defects.[20,21] Dr. Louis Elias, Pediatric Professor in Genetics at Emory University, tells us that the phenylalanine concentrates in the placenta, causing mental retardation.[22] Other researchers have warned from animal studies that aspartame, especially if used along with monosodium glutamate (MSG—another neurotoxin), may increase the likelihood of brain damage in children.[23,24]

With soda vending machines in many schools today, and with soft drinks containing aspartame becoming commonplace in countless households, one cannot help but speculate that there may be a connection between aspartame consumption and the seemingly increasing rates of autism and attention deficit hyperactive syndrome (ADHD) in children. Although ADHD is probably multifactoral, today's high intake of neurotoxins, like fluoride and aspartame, cannot be ruled out as a contributing factor. Although some studies indicate that aspartame may not greatly affect children who are already diagnosed with this condition, the question remains: How did they get that way in the first place? There is good reason to take a closer look at aspartame as a culprit.[25]

BETTY IS NOT ALONE

It is not just one activist, Betty Martini, who is making the claims against aspartame. There are dozens and dozens of respected scientists and researchers who have voiced their concerns about the dangers of this additive. Dr. George Schwartz, toxicologist, claims: "There is overwhelming scientific evidence that NutraSweet™ can pose a serious health threat."[26] Add to this list dozens of doctors who have improved their patients' health simply be telling them to remove aspartame from their diets. Beyond this anecdotal evidence is a recent study demonstrating how fibromyalgia symptoms disappeared by eliminating MSG and aspartame from the diet.[27] Research has also linked aspartame with headaches, including migraines.[28,29]

What about those concerned about weight gain? Isn't that why many people consume it in the first place? There is no evidence that consuming aspartame in place of sugar helps reduce weight. In fact, the American Cancer Society has noted that those who use artificial sweeteners gain more weight than those who don't use them. There is evidence that not only is aspartame addictive,[30] but that it also stimulates the appetite,[31,32] creating in the body a condition that craves carbohydrates in its sudden desire for more calories.

Aspartame may also be responsible for weight gain by virtue of its effect on chromium. This is a mineral in which many Americans are deficient. Such a deficiency has been linked to diabetes and its precursor—Syndrome X—in which a person can experience decreased HDL levels, insulin resistance, high blood pressure, and obesity. Chromium (meat, shellfish, chicken, cheese, unrefined grains, brewer's yeast) helps to regulate sugar and insulin levels and may be of use in preventing this prediabetic condition—and be an aid in weight control. One of the elements in aspartame (aspartic acid) is said to bind, or chelate, with chromium.[33]

If this process effectively removes chromium from the body, then it is clear that aspartame should never be recommended for diabetics.

FDA AT IT AGAIN

How could such an additive ever get approval from the FDA in the first place? Well, it took a long time (16 years) because the animal studies conducted by the manufacturer (Searle) were troublesome. The brain tumor rate for test animals was so high that FDA scientists and statisticians fought against approval. It was also noticed that some of the studies submitted by Searle were fraudulent; some of the lab tests were faked and the dangers concealed.[34] One FDA toxicologist working at that time, Dr. Adrian Gross, testified before the U.S. Congress that aspartame was capable of producing brain tumors.[35]

Most scientists at the FDA were not pleased, to say the least. In fact, The FDA Chief Counsel recommended that a grand jury investigate Searle for "falsifying animal studies conducted to establish the safety of aspartame."[36] The case, however, never came to trial. Government investigators caused one delay after another. According to Erik Millstone, a researcher at Sussex University, a particular U.S. Attorney, who was given the task of bringing fraud charges against the aspartame manufacturer, took a position with Searle's law firm, letting the statute of limitations run out.[37]

Searle (later purchased by Monsanto) was off the hook. And then came along a Reagan appointee, the new commissioner of the FDA, Arthur Hull Hayes, Jr. In 1980 an FDA Board of Inquiry voted unanimously against the approval of aspartame, but in 1981 Hayes put himself in position to overrule them. Just like that, after eight years of refusing to approve aspartame's use, this additive was declared safe for dry goods. Two years later he and his assistant gave the approval for the use of aspartame in soft drinks.

Two months after that, Commissioner Hayes left office for another job. That's right. A UPI investigative reporter found that he took a job with Searle's public relations firm at a reported salary of $1000 per day.[38] It would be of interest to know what Searle got in the way of subsequent work from Mr. Hayes since it was reported that he refused to talk to the press for years afterward—odd for a PR man. On the other hand, Searle could probably afford to pay him such a nice salary because his decisions to approve aspartame later generated billions of dollars in sales worldwide for the NutraSweet™ industry. Its product can be found today in over 5000 different items.

CORRUPTION AT THE FDA

Four other FDA officials connected with the approval of aspartame took positions with its manufacturer between 1979 and 1982. Such collusion between government and industry is, of course, not uncommon. According to the November 1992 *Townsend Letter for Doctors*, 37 of 49 top FDA officials who left the FDA took positions with companies they had regulated, and 150 FDA officials owned stock in drug companies they were assigned to manage. Who's guarding the hen house?

Companies without the deep pockets of Monsanto don't seem to fare quite as well with the FDA. Take the producers of stevia, for example. Stevia is a natural herbal sweetener. It cannot be patented. It has an excellent track record of safety. It is used freely in several countries. And it would be perfect for diabetics because of its positive effect on blood sugar. How did the FDA respond to stevia? They barred it from import in 1991—presumably because it would take away too much in the way of sales from NutraSweet™. Today, however, stevia is permitted into the United States—only as a food supplement though—not as a food additive like aspartame. The big money is still being protected.

Although approval of aspartame clearly violated the Delaney Clause, which prohibits the addition of substances shown to be carcinogenic in food, there appears to be no one around to police the FDA. A former FDA investigator left because of the shady practices he witnessed. On the matter of aspartame, he was told to keep his mouth shut.[39] He has publicly stated that the FDA seemed to be in collusion with corporations marketing substances detrimental to public health.

THE RESEARCH CONTINUES

Thanks to people like Betty Martini, the truth is getting out. Her critics have nothing to hide behind except their tired statements that "hundreds of studies have been conducted attesting to the safety of aspartame." What are those studies? They are the ones paid for by Searle and Monsanto.

Dr. Ralph Walton, Chairman of the Center for Behavioral Medicine at Northeastern Ohio University's College of Medicine, has shown that virtually all the studies showing the safety of aspartame were funded by the industry.[40] He produces evidence that when all of the industry studies are tossed out, as well as those with FDA involvement, what's left is a collection of independent studies—83 in total. Every single one of them shows adverse reactions to aspartame.

Three years after Ms. Martini created a firestorm with her revelations in 1995, one more very important bit of research damning aspartame came to light. Work conducted at the University of Barcelona tracked ingested aspartame as it broke down into DNA-damaging formaldehyde. They proved that it was stored in tissue and organs, including the brain, building up stores of this toxin. They modestly concluded that "aspartame consumption may constitute a hazard because of its contribution to the formation of formaldehyde."[41]

It has subsequently been reported that these researchers are now frightened after having received threats concerning their work.[42]

■■ **TIPS:** ■■

If you suffer from migraines or fibromyalgia symptoms, try eliminating all aspartame and MSG from your diet.

Since nearly all "diet" or "sugar free" products contain a harmful sugar substitute, opt for raw honey, maple syrup, molasses, or stevia.

OSTEOPOROSIS

Propaganda: Hormone Replacement Therapy (HRT) stops bone loss. We must increase our bone density. Everyone needs to drink milk because of calcium's role in maintaining good bone health.

Reality: HRT in no way helps to improve bone density and can increase the risk of dementia, stroke, and blood clots. Calcium is only one of the many nutrients needed for good bone health.

More Than Just calcium

We often seek simple answers to nutritional questions. The simplest and most obvious, the better. For instance, if cholesterol blocks coronary arteries, then the solution is to stop eating so many cholesterol-rich foods.

Well, we now know the problem is more complex. Dietary cholesterol seems to play an insignificant role in the development of heart disease. Just ask the heart-healthy Eskimos. Likewise, the simple answer given to the question of how to stop osteoporosis—eat more calcium-rich foods or, for menopausal women, take estrogen—is another example of straight-line thinking that can result in dangers to health.

Industries hoping to profit from this kind of simplistic approach certainly contribute to the problem. Pharmaceutical companies have for years been telling doctors and the women they treat that hormone replacement therapy (HRT) is what they need to stop the loss of bone, or Fosamax™, which in the short term creates denser bones, but in the long term leads to weaker ones.[1] And the milk industry says, as we have heard, that everybody needs milk. Problem solved. Wrong.

Osteoporosis, the extreme thinning of the bones that contributes to higher rates of fracture, can be said to have its beginning in humans after they turn 30. At that time, more bone seems to be lost than is replaced, and the problem accelerates at menopause. Bone, of course, is living tissue which is constantly changing. Over time, however, if a great decline in bone mineral density (BMD) occurs, then bone health is compromised. Right? Well, yes and no.

Standard Treatments

The Japanese have lower BMD than Americans, but they have lower rates of fracture.[2–4] Simply put, they have healthier bones despite the lower density. So to suggest to menopausal women that what they need is more estrogen to slow bone loss, is a dangerous proposition because of the increased risk of breast cancer associated with hormone replacement therapy (HRT).[5,6] Also, women are currently being warned about the increased risk of dementia, blood clots, stroke, and heart disease from HRT, even though they were earlier told HRT was just what they needed to protect the heart.

Some studies suggest that estrogen plays only a minor role in slowing bone loss; it is estimated that 30 percent of postmenopausal women do not lose significant amounts of bone.[7] And estrogen in no way helps to improve bone density. According to hormone and fluoride expert, Dr. John Lee, estrogen can only slow the rate of bone loss for a few years during menopause.[8] After that, it is ineffective. Is it worth the risks then?

If unpleasant symptoms of menopause cannot be controlled naturally with stress reduction or with the use of the herb maca, vitex, milk thistle, bioflavonoids, and vitamin E, then estriol, the "forgotten estrogen," might be considered.[9] It appears to be much safer than standard HRT and seems to display anticancer activity.

In terms of actually increasing bone density and helping to alleviate other menopausal symptoms, Dr. Lee suggests the use of natural progesterone. A carefully monitored use of small amounts of this hormone appears to have no untoward side effects. By raising the body's levels of progesterone—which decline to a greater extent at menopause than does estrogen—hormonal balance is restored, "estrogen dominance" disappears, and bone density increases. Although there is obvious value in increasing bone density, it must be remembered that the quality of the bone is as important as its density. Care must be taken to maintain the integrity of this newly gained bone mass.

Lessons were learned from the use of sodium fluoride, despite its toxicity, as a medical means to increase bone density: The quality of the bone, though dense, turned out to be inferior, resulting in very brittle bones. And, of course, the elderly, who have lived for many years in communities that artificially fluoridate their water, have higher rates of hip fractures.

Another popular remedy for osteoporosis is the synthetic soy isoflavone called ipriflavone. Like fluoride, it has been reported to help increase bone density. However, some research has shown it to be ineffective for this purpose. What's worse is that many of the women using this supplement have shown reduced white blood cell counts which returned to normal after discontinuing its use.[10] Save your money on this one.

SLOWING AND REVERSING BONE LOSS

Rather than focusing our attention too greatly on bone density, perhaps we should consider overall bone health, as well as the factors that contribute to an accelerated rate of bone loss. Losing too much bone mass, particularly at menopause, is a real concern for many. So what nutritional and lifestyle changes can be made to make certain that the loss is as slow as possible, while retaining strong, healthy bones?

We don't have to mention exercise, do we? We've heard it before. We know the value. Exercise can prevent and even reverse bone loss. Surprisingly, even the nonweight-bearing activity of swimming has proven to strengthen the bones. But are we committed to getting the exercise necessary for stronger bones? As Americans continue to become a more sedentary culture, the rate of bone fractures is sure to climb. There is a glimmer of hope with certain women, however, who are realizing that it's okay to have some muscle definition—or even some soft curves. A note to women: Some men appreciate some muscle on women—provided it's not greater than their own. And some like a more rounded figure. Both body types are better for the bones. With more muscle mass (since muscle weighs more than fat) the bones become stronger by virtue of the work they are required to do. This is perhaps the reason men develop osteoporosis much less often than women; they have more body mass. And since men do indeed develop this disease, this further demonstrates that osteoporosis is not tied solely to estrogen deficiency.

Beyond exercise, it is important to eat a nutrient-dense diet of unrefined foods that supply all the necessary factors to promote healthy bone tissue. Much more than just calcium is required. Consider these facts: Countries whose populations consume the largest amounts of calcium-rich dairy products (United States, Sweden, Finland, Canada, France, etc.) have the greatest incidence of osteoporosis.[11] And in the population with the least amount of osteoporosis, the Bantu of Africa, their average daily calcium intake of 325 mg. is less than a third of what we deem essential, but they have the same bone density.[12,13] In such cultures with strong bones, where the calcium intake is considered low, they are consuming foods, particularly vegetables, that supply the other nutrients necessary for bone health: essential fatty acids, zinc, copper, boron, manganese, silicon, vitamin K (found in leafy greens, egg yolks, and legumes, and which is depleted by the use of antibiotics), and especially magnesium and potassium.

ESSENTIAL MINERALS

Potassium appears to slow down the rate at which calcium is excreted from the body and also seems to increase the rate of new bone formation. And with magnesium, some research has suggested that proper levels of magnesium may be at least, if not more important, than calcium intake. Magnesium is necessary for the body to take calcium from the blood and lay it down in the bones. Too much calcium in the absence of magnesium, instead, can result in calcification of body tissues including artery walls. Yes, too much calcium in certain forms can be a problem, as evidenced by populations heavily consuming dairy without the complementary nutrients to help assimilate the calcium—nutrients like vitamin D and saturated fat (as 50 percent of the total fat intake[14]). Since intake of saturated fat is crucial for assimilation of calcium, it is less useful to consume only nonfat milk. Milk, however, doesn't seem to have enough magnesium to properly balance the calcium, so attention needs to be paid to obtaining more of this mineral for proper balance.[15–17]

Keeping in mind that stress and alcohol deplete your stores of magnesium, it is wise to add, for example, magnesium-rich almonds to your yogurt, or supply your needs with the additional magnesium found in beans, nuts, whole grain cereals, seafoods, and dark green vegetables. It has been suggested that magnesium and calcium should be consumed on a one to one basis.

A healthy-functioning thyroid is essential for strong bones, making hypothyroidism a risk factor for osteoporosis. The hypothyroid crisis in the United States (likely due in part to too much fluoride and too much unfermented soy consumption) is influenced by an insufficient availability of another important mineral: iodine. This mineral supports the thyroid and may in part explain less bone fractures among the Japanese: They have a good supply of iodine from the fish and sea vegetables they consume. In addition, a plentiful supply of vitamin K present in the diet of many Japanese (as found in fermented soy products) appears to offer protection against osteoporosis.[18] Soy products per se seem to be of little value in terms of achieving greater bone density.[19]

ANIMAL PROTEIN

But before we solve all of our problems with these added nutrients, we must consider what we are doing wrong to accelerate bone loss. This may turn out to be the most crucial issue of all, and it is not, as some would have us believe, simply that we are consuming too much animal protein, including that which is found in milk.

As noted, countries with high intakes of dairy also have high rates of osteoporosis. The antimilk and antimeat lobby maintains that the problem is too much acid-forming animal protein, which draws calcium from the bones. Some have just said flat-out that milk causes osteoporosis. What they may be overlooking is the fact that many of those countries consuming the highest amounts of dairy also have the highest percentages of people living past the age of 65. Therefore, we are naturally going to see more cases of osteoporosis. Plus, to confuse the issue, rates of osteoporosis seem to be on the rise in the United States even though milk consumption today is half of what it was in 1945. Some, however, have argued that the incidence of osteoporosis has not risen as much as we have been led to believe. Rather, it may be our definition of what constitutes osteoporosis that has changed. By relying solely on BMD readings, we have classified more people as being at risk. We have created a broader field for a disease that the pharmaceutical companies are quite eager to exploit. Regardless, factors other than milk are certainly involved with high rates of osteoporosis in many developed countries.

In Scandinavian countries where high dairy consumption matches high rates of osteoporosis, they also consume very high amounts of vitamin A, not only from fortified milk, but also from fish oils. High amounts of vitamin A are associated with high rates of osteoporotic fractures[20,21]—particularly when, according to clinical nutritionist Krispin Sullivan, large amounts of this vitamin are not balanced with enough vitamin D, which is also essential for the proper use of calcium in the body. Too much A can create a D deficiency.

To blame osteoporosis on milk is not fair in view of the fact that so much of the Scandinavian population is already vitamin-D deficient, especially during the winter months at these high latitudes. This is true for many Canadians as well.[22] With a paucity of sunlight, the production of vitamin D on the skin cannot match the otherwise healthful intakes of vitamin A. Balance is thrown off. And vitamin D from sunlight is more useful in promoting bone health than that which comes from supplements.[23] It is interesting to note that, unlike their continental counterparts, Caucasians living in Hawaii have low hip fracture rates like the Japanese who live both in Hawaii and in Japan.[24] It must be all that sun and fish (and less fluoridated water). Not only is there evidence that vitamin D may reduce the risk of death from heart disease, it has been shown that those getting the most ultraviolet-B from sunlight at lower latitudes are less likely to get thirteen different types of cancers.[25] Vitamin D is very underappreciated.

BACK TO THE PROTEIN

To be fair, animal protein like that found in milk can, in very high amounts, rob calcium from the bones. But how? It has to do with the pH balance in the body. Most bodily systems seem to work best in a slightly alkaline environment and are therefore better able to resist disease. The blood, for example, prefers a pH of about 7.4. Anything less than that results in the blood being too acidic, which can lead to a loss of muscle mass and reduced hormone levels. Plus, the body tries to compensate by pulling calcium from the bones to buffer the excess acid.

Animal protein is one food source that contributes to this acidity. Our early ancestors, however, typically ate greater quantities of animal protein than we do without resulting in bone problems because they had huge alkaline mineral reserves from the other food they consumed. A high intake of animal protein, including milk, need not be a problem provided the diet is otherwise adequate. In fact, a low protein intake has been found to result in greater bone loss in the elderly.[26,27] Milk and animal protein are not enemies of strong bones when they get the support of a nutrient-rich diet that includes plenty of alkaline foods.

OSTEOPOROSIS AND VEGETARIANS

The foods that are alkaline-forming and counteract an acid build-up are, as you may have guessed, most fruits and vegetables. We would assume, then, that vegetarians have greater bone density than their meat and dairy-consuming counterparts. This is not necessarily the case. Recent studies have demonstrated that a diet higher in animal protein, especially dairy (not vegetable protein), contributes to less fractures and greater bone density in certain age groups.[28,29] Though lowered bone mineral density is not always a sign of increased chances of fracture, recent studies have shown groups of vegetarians, especially vegans, to have less BMD than their meat-eating counterparts.[30,31] How can this be?

Well, animal-based foods are not the only acid-forming ones. Pasta, beans, lentils, legumes, nuts (except almonds), and most grains, including wheat and rice, are all acid-forming (unless sprouted). Vegetarians who rely heavily on these staples may unwittingly create an acid environment that rivals the big meat eaters, and are likely to accelerate bone loss. In addition, vegetarians who do not obtain enough vitamin D from sunlight, which aids in calcium absorption, may not be getting enough from a diet that does not include eggs, fish, and dairy. A diet too high in vegetable foods that contain significant amounts of mineral-binding substances—phytates and oxalates—can further contribute to bone problems for vegetarians.

The correct ratio of alkaline-forming foods to the acid ones is generally regarded as four to one. But how many of us still refuse to eat the necessary fruits and veggies to maintain this balance? Simply cutting out most protein and all acid-forming foods is not the best strategy because of the tremendous wealth of nutrients in these foods. Also, adequate amounts of protein, including dairy sources, can assist in the production of healthy bones for children, the middle-aged, and the elderly.[32-34] The large Nurses Health Study showed that only very large amounts of animal protein were capable of resulting in increased rates of bone fractures.[35] Incidentally, the same researchers did find in a 2003 study that total calcium intake was not associated with hip fracture risk, but it was adequate vitamin D that was protective in postmenopausal women.[36] It appears that we may need plenty of protein to protect our bones more than we need the calcium, and of course, we need the D or sunlight to utilize what calcium we do consume.

BONE ROBBERS

So what else could be drawing calcium from the bones besides a diet that is too acid? Look no further than the usual list of culprits: tobacco, caffeine (notably coffee which is also acid-forming), soft drinks, large amounts of sugar, and common, refined table salt (affecting those with high blood pressure[37]). All of these draw calcium from the bones and can contribute to osteoporosis. Perhaps the worst offenders are canned colas.

We don't have to go into the statistics. You know the story. Teenage girls, especially, are drinking way too much cola and other soft drinks, which are replacing the very nutrients needed to create a reservoir of healthy bone tissue to last throughout a lifetime. For many children, soft drinks have largely replaced milk in their households, and today's kids often spend less time outdoors reaping the benefit of sunlight. Consequently, they aren't building enough bone in the first place and, in the second place, caffeine and sugar provide a potent calcium-draining, one–two punch. Sugar-free sodas, of course, are not an option because of the negative health effects of aspartame.

What's worse is that there is too much phosphorus in these drinks, as well as in many processed meats. Although phosphorous works with calcium to create healthy bones, too much of it upsets the balance and acts to draw calcium from the skeleton. Add this to the fact that aluminum from the cans leaches into the liquid and may further lead to weakened bones[38]—not to mention its association with the development of Alzheimer's disease. And oh, yes, most colas are produced with fluoridated water, which is already overconsumed in this country, leading to brittle bones and other serious maladies.

PLAIN AND SIMPLE

As a society, we are our own worst enemy when it comes to the health of our bones. If the Bantu culture can maintain healthy bones on minimal amounts of calcium, and if the Mayan women can typically live for twenty or more years past menopause without osteoporosis[39,40] (and without HRT), then perhaps American women can as well.

Bone fractures are not inevitable. With the right diet, we can do something about the strength of our bone architecture, which is at least as important as its density. Bone expert Susan E. Brown states, "Osteoporosis by itself does not cause bone fractures. This is documented by the fact that half of the population with thin osteoporotic bones in fact never fractures."[41]

So start balancing your pH levels by loading up on the vegetables and begin to limit the use of grains (except perhaps nonacid-forming millet and quinoa). Add other high-alkaline foods to the diet like figs, apricots, raisins (organic), green vegetables or powders, vegetable and bone broths, and even citrus juices and apple cider vinegar whose natural acids are converted to an alkaline state in the body. The alkaline properties of apple cider vinegar may by the key reason why it has such a wonderful healing reputation in folk-medicine lore. Remember, however, to limit the use of dried fruits because of their highly concentrated sugar content.

Improved pH will keep the calcium where it belongs and permit the digestive enzymes, which were once inhibited by an acid environment, to become fully functional and thereby allow the body to better absorb bone-healthy nutrients. Such nutrients include not only those mentioned so far, but also the essential fatty acids like the omega-3s and evening primrose oil,[42] and of course vitamin E, which protects the bones from oxidative damage that can result from a high consumption of refined vegetable oils.[43]

MORE RECOMMENDATIONS

Although there is some disagreement about whether milk products are acid or alkaline-forming, most seem to be close to neutral (except for some high-acid hard cheeses). It is quite likely that the high quality, raw, and/or organic milk products tend toward the alkaline side while supplying plenty of calcium for those who do not have milk allergies or are lactose intolerant. Regular supermarket milk should be avoided by everyone because the homogenization process facilitates the entrance of an enzyme called xanthine oxidase into the bloodstream where it is suspected of damaging the arterial walls, leading to cardiovascular disease, whose rates are high in those countries consuming lots of homogenized milk.

Also implicated in the development of osteoporosis, as well as heart disease, are high levels of the nonessential amino acid homocysteine.

Increasing intakes of the B vitamins, including folic acid, help to lower homocysteine levels.

Full-fat (organic) dairy products do not need to be avoided. Low-fat dairy is likely to have a higher acid profile because of the higher percentage of protein it contains. Furthermore, whole-milk products contain greater amounts of the healthy fatty acid conjugated linoleic acid (CLA). As we now know, this substance is found in beef and milk and is found in even greater amounts in animals that have been allowed to graze on green grass. CLA appears to build muscle mass, prevent hardening of the arteries, and offer cancer protection. What a deal!

For those not consuming dairy or who cannot entirely give up their bad habits, dietary or otherwise, eating plenty of dark, leafy greens, broccoli, nuts, and seeds is a must. If necessary, adding calcium supplements that are supported with plenty of magnesium might be a smart idea, as well as vitamin D, of course, for those unable to get out in the sunshine. But remember, too much unbalanced calcium can result in kidney stones and calcification of the soft tissues.

Despite the incomplete picture presented by those primed to benefit financially from our fear of thinning bones—the drug companies—the problem appears not to be so complex after all. Get exercise and sunlight; eat unrefined, nutrient-dense foods; do your best to reduce stress; and be conscious of your pH balance. Don't be fooled by the pharmaceutical companies. Your bones will thank you.

■■ **TIPS:** ■■

Exercise to increase bone strength.

For menopausal symptoms, supplement with vitex, the herb maca, milk thistle, bioflavonoids, and vitamin E.

For bone health, supplement with essential fatty acids, magnesium (found in almonds and other nuts, beans, seafood, and dark green vegetables), vitamin K (found in leafy, green vegetables), and potassium.

BOVINE GROWTH HORMONE

Propaganda: Monsanto's Bovine Growth Hormone (rBGH) produces milk that is as safe as naturally produced milk.

Reality: Increased milk production causes a rise in udder infections in cows, which can produce pus that collects in our milk along with antibiotics and IGF-1, an insulinlike hormone associated with cancer. Every other country in the world prohibits use of rBGH. In Germany, vets refuse to administer it on the grounds that it is cruel to cows.

(SOME) MILK IS NOT FOR ANYBODY

Nutrition pioneer Weston Price would be appalled to see what has happened to today's dairy products. He had given strong evidence of the health-giving potential of milk from grass-fed animals. But with much of today's milk pasteurized and homogenized, containing traces of pesticides and antibiotics, we have a product that is anything but healthy.

How about a little pus in your milk? That, plus something worse (if you can imagine that), is what you are likely to get as a result of the newest assault on a once healthy product. The travesty now being perpetrated on the milk-drinking public is the use of Monsanto's genetically engineered bovine growth hormone, rBGH (also called rBST).

Despite an oversupply of milk for which the dairy industry is subsidized by taxpayers, costing us more than $200 million dollars each year,[1] some dairy farmers want even greater milk production. Who can blame them since they benefit from price supports and the government's willingness to buy the surplus? Consequently, many farmers have turned to the use of rBGH, which speeds up a cow's metabolism, creating longer lactation periods and more milk.

Apparently, the farmers who inject their herds with this stuff are not overly concerned about the welfare of the animals. By artificially stimulating milk production, the individual cow's life is reported by many farmers to be shortened by an average of two years. And during this shortened lifespan, the cows suffer reproductive problems, lameness from hoof problems, and increased instances of mastitis, an udder infection that can result in pus being added to the collected milk.[2,3] The sickened cows are then subjected to more antibiotics, which can find their way into the milk and into the consuming public. This ultimately can lead to the ever-increasing problem of bacterial resistance to existing antibiotics.

Veterinarians in Germany, however, play by a more humane set of rules. There, the vets refuse to administer rBGH on the grounds that it violates their code of ethics, which forbids intentional animal cruelty.[4]

LIES FROM THE FDA

It is clear that this added hormone harms the cows, but what about the people who drink their milk? The FDA, which gave approval to rBGH in 1993, said that Monsanto's product was no different from the natural BGH already present in cow's milk and that it would have no specific impact on humans. Untrue. BGH acts as a growth hormone only in cows, we were told; the extra hormones in milk from injected cows would not be absorbed into the bloodstream. False, again.

The problem for people may not be the rBGH per se, but rather what it does inside the cow: rBGH creates elevated levels of another hormone called IGF-1 (insulinlike growth factor), which occurs naturally in the human body and is useful for a variety of metabolic functions. One study showed a sixfold increase of IGF-1 in milk from cows injected with rBGH.[5] Elevated amounts of IGF-1, however, are of great concern. It must be remembered that hormones are unlike many drugs in that they are extremely powerful in small amounts and can set up an entire chain of events in the human body.

The IGF-1 from milk is identical to that found in humans and is not destroyed by pasteurization; nor is it destroyed in the human stomach. It is absorbed into the bloodstream, thereby raising levels of this potent hormone, which causes cells to divide. The concern, of course, is with high amounts of IGF-1 and its ability to promote cancer.

MORE CANCER-CAUSING AGENTS IN THE FOOD CHAIN

The British journal *Lancet* reported a sevenfold increase in the risk of breast cancer in premenopausal women with the highest levels of IGF-1 in their blood.[6] The publication *Science* reported a fourfold increased risk of prostate cancer in men with elevated levels of IGF-1, even though these levels were within the normal range.[7,8] This growth hormone has also been implicated in cancers of the lung and colon.[9] It is interesting to note that elevated levels of IGF-1 are also caused by consumption of fluoride[10] and soy protein.[11] British researchers have cautioned against consuming substances that increase concentrations of IGF-1 because of "the increasing evidence of the risk of cancer."[12]

Dr. Michael Hansen, a researcher at the Consumer Union in New York, believes that the risk of polyps and tumors from IGF-1 in treated milk, along with an inadequate or improper evaluation of its safety by the FDA, is enough to pull rBGH off the market.[13] In fact, every other country in the world prohibits its use. The IGF-1 in treated milk is absorbed in the GI tract and is more bioactive than that in regular milk; these properties are enhanced by pasteurization.[14]

Dr. Samuel S. Epstein at the University of Illinois in Chicago is an expert on the environmental causes of cancer and has frequently been called upon to give expert testimony before Congress. He claims that the IGF-1 from rBGH-treated milk may well promote cancer of the breast and colon. He adds, "In short, with the active complicity of the FDA, the entire nation is being subjected to an experiment . . . it (rBGH) poses a major potential public health risk for the entire U.S. population."[15] With the clear health risks to cows and the potential for rBGH to cause human tumors, how could the FDA have ever granted approval to market this drug? Did the long period of testing on animals before approval reveal no risks at all? Well, the FDA has kept these details under wraps.

You see, a key 90-day study on 30 rats conducted by Monsanto, which convinced the FDA to approve their drug, has never been made public—or even made available to the independent scientific community. Monsanto and the FDA refuse to reveal the results. If the results were released, the FDA claims it would "irreparably harm Monsanto."[16] What? Is it the FDA's job to protect Monsanto or is it to inform and protect the public?

SOUND SCIENCE IGNORED

Interestingly, most studies that test a new drug's long-term potential last for two years and involve hundreds of animals. Why the FDA relied heavily of a 90-day study is most curious indeed.

When details of this linchpin study finally began to leak out during rBGH's approval process in Canada, it was discovered that several serious problems existed. Some of the rats tested had developed cysts. Some developed antibodies to the rBGH. This should have raised a red flag.[17] The FDA gave approval anyway. When confronted with this information, the FDA responded by saying that it never got the precise data from the study. All they had was a summary from Monsanto. How can approval be granted when the raw data from the most important study is not examined by a team of scientists? Such conduct violates their own regulations. Something is very wrong.

It appears, once again, that the FDA and Monsanto were working as a team. Approval seems to have been a done-deal from the beginning. An FDA branch chief involved in the rBGH approval process had been previously employed for four years by Monsanto to oversee their rBGH studies. The summary she signed off on, and which formed the basis for

FDA approval of this hormone, made no mention of the 90-day study that clearly showed serious problems. It only referred to a 28-day study that concluded: "No adverse effects were observed in test animals."[18] Apparently, the term "conflict of interest" is something that is ignored at the FDA.

CANADA GETS INVOLVED

The pressure from Monsanto to get widespread acceptance of its product was great north of the border as well. Health Canada, the Canadian counterpart to the FDA, was applying pressure to their own scientists to quickly approve rBGH. According to a program aired on CBC-TV, scientists there reported bribes of $1-2 million offered by Monsanto to approve rBGH without further testing.[19] Monsanto denies this, saying that the money was offered for research purposes. One wonders how the money could be used for "research" if Monsanto wanted quick approval.

Like the FDA, Health Canada was secretive about the now famous 90-day study. A few scientists there, however, demanded to see the specifics of the research done by Monsanto. They found data missing from FDA records. They found that the report falsely claimed that rBGH could not be absorbed in the blood. They were disturbed by what appeared to be rBGH's link to prostate and thyroid disorders and to certain types of cancer. What they found resulted in a paper subsequently written by them known as the "Gaps Analysis" which found errors, omissions, and other faults with the study. With regard to the accuracy of this key study, the Canadian scientists concluded: ". . . such possibilities and potentials as sterility, infertility, birth defects, cancer and immunological derangements were not addressed."[20]

This report led to the formation of two Canadian panels of researchers to address the safety of rBGH. The first panel was to look at human health concerns and the second was to study animal safety. According to the *Toronto Star*, among the members of the first panel was a former Monsanto employee, a physician who had served as a consultant to Monsanto and had published a paper recommending that the Canadian government approve rBGH.[21,22] Predictably, the panel found little wrong with the Monsanto product, except for elevated levels of IGF-1. The second team, however, found enough convincing evidence of harm to cows that rBGH was, after nine years of study, rejected in 1999. Evidently, the influence of Monsanto is not quite as great in Canada as it is in the United States.

TRUTH-TELLING IS RISKY

Back in the states, Fox TV in Tampa, Florida, fired two investigative reporters for trying to expose the truth about the possible dangers of rBGH. Award-winning reporters Steve Wilson and Jane Aker had been asked to produce a TV series on rBGH in milk. The series was stopped three days before airing after the station had received two threatening letters from Monsanto.

One letter cited the "enormous damage" Monsanto would incur if the program were shown. The other letter was more threatening. It claimed there would be "dire consequences" if the station proceeded with the reports.[23,24]

Management at the Fox station ordered the reporters to make changes to the series, particularly where it addressed cancer concerns. Steve and Karen would not consent to the changes. They were even offered money to leave the station and keep quiet about what the station was planning with their work. They declined and were fired.

Eventually, these courageous reporters sued Fox and won $425,000 in damages for their treatment. Hopefully, this award will make up for the wages they lost by taking a moral stand. They have, however, had a difficult time getting full-time employment in mainstream media since they were unjustly fired. Big industry has a very long reach.

DOES YOUR MILK HAVE rBGH?

Monsanto has been very concerned about the public's reaction and possible mistrust of their new cow drug. And so it is no surprise that a former Monsanto employee, who was rehired by the company after his tenure at the FDA, was responsible for writing regulations prohibiting food labels that would tell consumers whether or not they were getting rBGH-treated products.[25] Monsanto itself got into the act in 1994 by suing two milk processors for trying to label their products "BGH free," and was reported to have sent out about 2000 warning letters to other dairy processors and retailers.[26]

Today, consumers still have difficulty knowing whether their milk, cream, cheese, ice cream, cottage cheese, yogurt, and other dairy products are made from rBGH-treated cows. About 30 percent of all U.S. cows are injected with this hormone, and much of their milk is blended at processing plants with the milk from dairies not using it.

In some states, however, consumers can find labels stating that the milk or cheese is rBGH (or rBST) free. Look for those products. Demand those products. Or, request and buy only organically produced or raw milk products, particularly from dairies that allow their cows to graze on grass. (For the availability of raw milk in your area, go to www.rawmilk.com.)

For those able to consume dairy, there can be tremendous nutritional benefit not only from the calcium, but also from the fat-soluble vita-mins, protein, and conjugated linoleic acid (CLA). But for the typical homogenized milk found in supermarkets, with its rBGH, antibiotics, pesticide residues—and pus—forget it.

■■ TIPS: ■■

Drink organic BGH/BST-free, unhomogenized milk only—fresh and raw when possible.

Try raw goat and sheep's milk too!

EGGS

Propaganda: Eating eggs leads to heart disease: throw out the yolks!

Reality: In reality, eggs are high in choline and B_6, both of which are used to combat hardening of the arteries. Eggs are nutrient dense and contain all the amino acids, a vast array of minerals and vitamins, and antioxidants.

MORE GOOD CHOLESTEROL NEWS

One of the most misguided bits of nutritional advice followed by many Americans during recent years has been to use only the egg whites and toss out the yolks. Talk about a waste of natural resources! The yolk is the best part.

Yes, there is plenty of cholesterol in the yolk, but we now know that the cholesterol issue is mostly a bogus one. With regard to eggs, the last decade has provided plenty of research showing that in healthy individuals (i.e., those not diabetic or with a genetic tendency to mishandle dietary cholesterol) there is no evidence to suggest that eating eggs correlates to a greater incidence of heart disease.[1]

The American Heart Association (AHA) finally relented in the year 2000 and changed its dietary allowance for eggs from three a week to the equivalent of one per day, provided other sources of cholesterol were limited. Research shows, however, that as many as 14 per week have been shown not to raise cholesterol in any significant way.[2] In fact, consumption of as many as 24 eggs per week results in no significant differences in blood cholesterol levels (compared to eating 0–2 1/2).[3] It appears that dietary cholesterol is simply not related to the incidence of coronary heart disease.[4] It can be assumed, however, that the AHA felt it would lose too much face if it were to admit that its previous severe restrictions on egg consumption were more than a little off base. Reflecting the kind of scientific thinking that appears to go on in this organization, we have the following statement by the chair of the AHA Dietary Guidelines Committee: "When you don't have any real good answers in this business, you have to accept a few not so good ones as the next best thing."[5]

FEAR OF EGGS

When good nutritionists are asked what is one of the top myths that the public falls prey to, the "danger" of eating too many eggs stands near the top of the list. It is difficult to change public perception of eggs because the so-called hazard of consuming its cholesterol has been engraved into the public's consciousness for decades. Egg phobia still exists in most quarters. This is especially troubling for the elderly who often follow whatever recommendations the "authorities" suggest. They are depriving themselves of vital nutrients they may be deficient in—among them vitamin D and protein. The yolk has almost as much protein as the white. Instead, too many folks are discarding those nutrient-dense yolks, or resorting to egg substitutes which are 99 percent egg whites.

How did this all start? Well, once again it was very old and faulty research that created a bad image for eggs. According to nutritionist Ann Louise Gittleman, experiments conducted over 50 years ago by the Cereal Institute put eggs on the dangerous food list.[6] In their studies, rather than use fresh, whole, unprocessed eggs, the way they were intended to be eaten, the researchers use dried egg yolk powder—which is oxidized and quite harmful to the arteries. Remember, unoxidized cholesterol is harmless in a healthy diet, but when the cholesterol in foods is heated to very high temperatures, it begins to oxidize and become toxic. This problem is compounded immensely when, under high heat and pressure, powders of milk or egg yolk are produced. These substances are culprits in heart disease and should be avoided.

So eggs got a bad rap, which was perpetuated when the government's anticholesterol campaign kicked into high gear over thirty years ago with dietary restrictions on eggs proposed in 1972. Even the federal court system got in on the act; in 1976 it told an egg-sellers association to stop saying that eating eggs doesn't increase the risk of heart attacks— even though there was no proof to the contrary.[7] At that time, the government and food industry were responsible for circulating a number of nutritional myths. According to reporter and author Omar V. Garrison, the public was fed the following food propaganda: (1) that an ordinary American diet (with its highly processed foods) will supply all the nutrients essential for health, (2) that the value of food is not affected by the type of soil or fertilizers used, (3) that foods cannot be effectively used to treat diseases, conditions, or symptoms, and (4) that a deficiency in vitamins and minerals is not due to the storage, transportation, processing, or cooking of foods.[8]

It is clear that during the 1970s all this nonsense promulgated by government and food interests was designed to convince the public that factory food was healthful: no need to resort to food supplements—and little need to eat whole foods grown on healthy soils. By condemning eggs, a whole new market for egg substitutes was established: more profit for industry at the expense of public health.

Champion for Common Sense

A number of researchers and nutritionists, however, knew better. They knew that the FDA was holding hands with industry. They knew that degenerative diseases were becoming more rampant on a supposedly healthful American diet that was becoming filled with more and more processed foods. They knew that eggs were being used as a scapegoat to appease the public. We were supposed to be reassured that health authorities were doing something valuable to stem the tide of heart disease—something valuable like telling the public to limit consumption of yet another whole food, a food never properly identified as anything but healthful.

One such nutritionist was Carlton Fredericks who repeatedly kicked the shins of public health officials because of their failure to protect the nutritional health of the public. The authorities did not take kindly to his assertions made in print and on the air via his radio talk show. They responded. For two decades he found himself vilified by government press releases. He found himself slandered by poison-pen letters to academic institutions, as well as threatened and censored by the FDA, FTC, FCC, and the IRS.[9] The government simply did not want the public to hear his message that the quality of food in this country was contributing to disease. But he continued to speak his mind.

Thirty-eight years ago he gave us truthful and insightful information about eggs and cholesterol in his book *Food, Facts, and Fallacies*. He suggested then that elevated cholesterol levels might represent some sort of protective effect against some onslaught. How right he was. We now know that cholesterol levels rise during stressful conditions. The cholesterol appears to be trying to protect us from unhealthful conditions created by stress. What is of special interest is that cholesterol has been shown to act as a powerful antioxidant[10,11]—yes, one of the treasured antioxidants like vitamin C, E, and coenzyme Q10, all of which have been shown to have heart-protective effects.

Dr. Fredericks also noted that eggs are rich in choline and vitamin B_6; both had been used successfully in treating hardening of the arteries. These are two of the very nutrients that are now being used by many to control what we think is a serious threat to heart health: high levels of homocysteine. Another nutrient has recently been found to combat homocysteine—betaine, a vitaminlike substance that also aids in brain function and is found in whole grains, fish, beets, and some greens, with liver and eggs considered by some to be the best sources. Also, some research indicates that eating eggs may raise the levels of the protective HDL cholesterol (good, of course).[12] Other studies show that egg consumption can lower total cholesterol. This is an example of how whole foods like eggs are protective—but not processed, powdered, or pulverized eggs.

CHOLESTEROL ECONOMICS

Why was the public so gullible about the supposed danger of cholesterol—allowing eggs, the "king" of cholesterol, to be so vilified? It has been suggested that it was partly due to a backlash from the era's counterculture movement[13]—when overconsumption of rich foods was a symptom of an overindulgent society far removed from nature and from the "benefits" of brown rice in a vegetarian diet. Was it, perhaps, simply a manifestation of the American brand of Puritan-style guilt? Anything fatty, rich, and satisfying must by definition be sinful. Whatever the reason, and because the cause of heart disease was so elusive at the time, cholesterol and eggs were demonized. In lieu of sound scientific answers implicating cholesterol in heart disease, a scapegoat would suffice. The dictocrats had little evidence, but they needed an answer, even if it was wrong.

If traditional consumption of high-fat, high-cholesterol foods was to be made into a taboo, then producers of eggs, dairy, and meat were sure to cry foul. This is exactly what happened. Despite their protestations, these industries were left holding the bag. The grain and edible oil industries had more clout. Replacing cholesterol-rich foods with processed, polyunsaturated vegetable oils would bring huge profits to these powerful lobbies. It has been pointed out that selling a pound of soy or corn oil is much more lucrative than selling a pound of butter or lard.

Egg consumption in the United States reached its per capita high in 1945 at 402 eggs per year. The last decade has seen levels fall to around 235 eggs per year. Has a corresponding decrease in heart disease matched this declining use of eggs? Of course not. Heart disease rates rose while egg consumption declined. Instead of eating protective whole foods like eggs, we began to replace them with processed polyunsaturated oils and, worse, partially hydrogenated ones. These oils are now proving to result in a greater chance of developing not only heart disease but also cancer.

TOP EGG CONSUMERS

We are often told to emulate the Japanese diet because of their greater longevity and very low rates of heart disease. We are told to consume more soy, as they supposedly do. As the nutritional counterpart to the shoe-marketing phrase "Be like Mike," we now have "Eat like Shinjo." Eat like the Japanese and be healthy.

However, the Japanese eat much less soy than many "health conscious" Americans. Soy milk consumption in Japan is insignificant (Saio, 1999), although its use seems to be growing. Many Japanese are now asking for soy milk in their cafe lattes. Perhaps they are trying to emulate Americans by using this product, while Americans consume soy milk thinking they are emulating the Japanese!

The Japanese do, however, eat more eggs than Americans. They love eggs. In fact, they consume more eggs per person than any nation in the world.[14] They regard eggs as a brain food. Could it be a heart food as well? The nutritional experts who advise us to eat more soy for the heart, by the same logic, should advise Americans to eat more eggs like the Japanese. What an interesting concept—more eggs, less heart disease. This, however, is not a very politically correct notion. A favorite study concerning eggs and cholesterol was reported in the medical journal *Metabolism*, and paraphrased by Dr. David Reuben in his classic book *Everything You Always Wanted to Know About Nutrition*:

> Half the subjects were confined to bed because they were sick, and the other half were normal people like the rest of us. All the participants were given the equivalent of nine eggs a day—more than the average person eats, to be sure. At the end of the study period only two of the sick people showed any elevation in cholesterol—and they'd had trouble in that area before. After eating their nine eggs every day, the healthy people had lower [total] cholesterol than when they started.[15]

A NUTRIENT TREASURE TROVE

OK, besides the high-quality protein, what else is so good about eggs? Ann Louise Gittleman points out that an egg is a germinative food—one that gives rise to a larger organism. Germinative foods like sprouts and seeds are among the most valuable because they are so nutrient-dense. In an egg, a rich source of nutrients must support the emerging chick. It appears that much of what supports the chick also supports human beings as well. That is, the egg contains all the amino acids as well as a vast array of the minerals and vitamins we need for health, with the exception of vitamin C, which the chick synthesizes on its own. In short, next to mother's milk (and very close to it) eggs have the best nutrient package of any food we can eat. It appears to be the healthiest staple food on the planet. The high fat and cholesterol content of mother's milk is known to give rise to a healthy infant brain. Therefore, to see very young children put on a low-fat diet borders on the criminal. They need the fat and cholesterol and so do we. Consider eggs the adult replacement for breast milk. (I do not work for the egg companies, if you are wondering. Really.)

Egg yolks also contain lecithin (high in choline), another brain-healthy nutrient, giving credence to the Japanese belief that they are indeed a "brain food." The brain is substantially composed of lecithin (and cholesterol). Lecithin helps to emulsify cholesterol and make its incorporation into the cells more efficient. In fact, the word "lecithin" derives from the Greek word for egg yolk, *lekithos.* Furthermore, lecithin is a prime component of the valuable HDL cholesterol, and this may be one reason why HDL levels have been shown to rise with egg consumption.

Besides being a good source of folate and vitamin A, eggs supply vitamins D and B_{12}, which are lacking in so many foods. Although not deemed essential, but nevertheless shown to be valuable antioxidants, are the carotenoids lutein and zeaxanthin. Green vegetables like spinach and broccoli are sources, besides eggs, which contain these nutrients thought to be especially helpful in helping to prevent cataracts and macular degeneration.

MISLED BY FRAMINGHAM

Critics of the premise that we should include cholesterol-rich foods into a healthy diet will point to the famous Framingham study, which did correlate high cholesterol levels with a greater incidence of heart disease (in younger men). Whether it was intentional or not, the early press releases from the Framingham study were incomplete and misleading. The public was convinced to avoid cholesterol in foods like the plague even though, as we know, dietary cholesterol has very little impact on levels in the blood and does not result in higher rates of heart disease. Important information contained in the study, and which was never released to the public, involved a subgroup of Framingham subjects specifically selected to focus on the impact of diet on blood cholesterol levels. The researchers concluded: "There is, in short, no suggestion of any relation between diet and the subsequent development of CHD (coronary heart disease) in the study group."[16] Who decided to withhold this information and why—as the anticholesterol forces continued to gain momentum?

Although there is a small segment of the population with a genetic condition known as familial hypercholesterolemia in which dietary cholesterol is not processed properly by the body, giving rise to very high LDL levels, it would be foolish to suggest that everyone with a cholesterol reading over 240 should be medicated to lower this number. About thirteen million Americans are taking these dangerous cholesterol-lowering medications, and this is particularly troubling for the elderly who are advised to do so. High cholesterol readings for the elderly appear not to be a risk factor for heart disease at all. In fact, it now seems that for the elderly, women in particular, higher readings may be protective and are associated with longevity.[17]

A DIGRESSION INTO THE WORLD OF DRUGS

With the current emphasis on consuming more polyunsaturated oil and less saturated fat and cholesterol, the edible oil companies are sitting pretty. And so, of course, are the drug companies who earn over $4 billion a year peddling their cholesterol drugs (statins). In fact, things recently got better for them when, in 2001, the government revised downward the cholesterol numbers used to determine whether a patient should be advised to take cholesterol-lowering medication. We can soon expect about 35 million Americans to be on these drugs. Something is very wrong. The message to cut back on cholesterol did little good in saving lives; now we are told that most cholesterol levels between 200 and 240 are no longer normal when HDL and LDL profiles are not acceptable according to the new guidelines. More people put on drugs. More profits for the drug companies. And no proof that these drugs provide any lasting, long-term benefit. In fact, researcher and nutritionist Robert Crayhon claimed in 1994 that statistics showed that these drugs will shorten your life.[18] Biochemist Udo Erasmus also notes greater suicide and cancer deaths among those who "indiscriminately" lower cholesterol as suggested by the National Educational Program. Apparently, the same LDL cholesterol, which medication is designed to reduce, also carries fat-soluble, anticancer antioxidants like vitamins A and E and beta carotene to the cells.[19]

All this makes you question how many drug company representatives were involved in setting the new guidelines—which they hope will eventually see half of the American population taking statins. (The answer: six.) Six of the "recognized experts" on the panel setting the new guidelines were reported to have received consultant fees from the makers of the statin drugs.[20] Drug company profits from these medications are expected to reach into the many billions of dollars.

Recent studies funded by these pharmaceutical corporations have shown that their statins greatly reduce cholesterol levels and, at least in the short term, decrease the incidence of heart attacks—but not nearly to the extent that drinking plenty of pure water does, as shown by the Loma Linda study. What has not been demonstrated is that the cholesterol drop precipitated by these drugs is what is responsible for the positive results. Statins have a number of pharmacological effects. Since these cholesterol-lowering medications seem to be effective even in people with already low cholesterol levels—people who theoretically should not be at risk—we suspect that it is one or more of the other biological effects of statins which are responsible for their short-term success. And there is some research to indicate that this is so.[21]

Recent studies concerning the causes of heart disease have focused on the role of chronic, painless inflammation caused by a simmering infection. Such inflammation, as evidenced by high levels of C-reactive protein, appears to be a much more potent marker for heart disease than high cholesterol levels. Instead of acting merely as a sign that there is something amiss in the body, this inflammation appears to participate in the disease process by virtue of the artery-damaging proteins it creates. Diet and exercise dramatically lower the effects of this inflammatory condition, and statins also reduce levels of these harmful proteins. This may be the very mechanism by which these drugs have short-term value—not because they lower levels of cholesterol. But what are the drawbacks of using statins as opposed to doing what makes sense—improving diet and exercising?

STATIN SIDE EFFECTS

The effects of statins give real cause for concern. Besides lowering cholesterol, they block the synthesis of CoQ10, a very important heart nutrient. In the long run, it is conceivable that by blocking this key nutrient more heart disease may be caused instead of prevented. Of course, that one percent of the population with a genetic tendency toward high cholesterol (hypercholesterolemia) may need these drugs, but it is recommended that they supplement their diet with CoQ10 to prevent further health problems.

We know that cholesterol is essential in maintaining cell membrane integrity. What would happen if there is a sudden and dramatic loss of cholesterol? Wouldn't we expect the cells to suffer? Two of the side effects of statins indicate that this is exactly what happens when cholesterol levels experience an unnatural decline.

Statins have been linked to a dangerous condition, especially for the elderly, called rhabdomyolysis. Those suffering from this ailment find their muscle cells breaking down, with the cell contents spilling into the bloodstream. This can lead to possible kidney failure and death. Because over 30 deaths were linked to the use of the statin Baycol™, this drug was removed from the market in 2001, although the maker of this product, Bayer, and its marketing partner, GlaxoSmithKline, are accused of marketing it even after having knowledge of deaths resulting from its use. The watchdog group Public Citizen has pointed out that over 80 additional rhabdomyolysis deaths have been associated with the use of other statins currently on the market. They have petitioned the FDA to warn doctors and patients about this deadly side effect.

OTHER STATIN CONCERNS

The highest concentration of cholesterol is in the brain and nervous system. Deprived of this nutrient, nerve cells may suffer. Researchers have suggested that lowering cholesterol levels with statins may have a toxic effect on the nerves. They found a 4–14 times increase in a particular form of nerve damage (polyneuropthy) in people taking statins for two or more years.[22] Polyneuropthy can result in permanent damage.

Besides depleting CoQ10, statins have been shown to cause liver dysfunction and to substantially reduce levels of beta carotene and vitamin E, antioxidants important in maintaining cardiovascular health, and they also appear to raise insulin levels.[23] Developing "insulin resistance" is an early sign of diabetes which, of course, contributes to a greater risk of heart disease.

How about cancer? Yes, statins have been shown to cause cancer in lab animals. The researchers who made these findings noted that the rodents got cancer in some cases "at levels of animal exposure close to those prescribed to humans." They recommended that statins "should be avoided except in patients at high short-term risk of cardiovascular disease."[24]

In humans, it may take quite a few years for cancer to develop from a specific initiator. Even so, there is evidence that treating women with statins may increase the risk of getting breast cancer—a risk that may be greater than the decreased risk of heart disease.[25] And in men it can cause erectile dysfunction. Statins have been identified as a culprit in "drug-induced impotence."[26] It is interesting to note that the makers of one of these popularly prescribed cholesterol-lowering medications also manufactures Viagra™.

The short-term benefits of statins, however, may outweigh the risks of some of the side effects—for a while. We just don't have a clue, though, about the long-term results of medicating perhaps 35 million Americans with drugs whose action on the cardiovascular system may have nothing to do with cholesterol reduction. If the value of these drugs has to do with decreasing inflammation in the heart, there are other safer tools to accomplish this. Critics of these statins have complained that the trials used to justify their approval were too small or too short. They may be right. A recent and larger study showed that use of the statin drug Pravastatin™ did not significantly reduce cardiovascular disease or all-cause mortality in users compared to "usual care" in older participants.[27]

This calls into question the validity of the earlier studies that were used to gain approval of these drugs. All of those statin trials were sponsored by the companies whose drugs were being tested.[28] A conflict of interest is possible. In fact, a review of the data finds that industry-sponsored studies were 3.6 times more likely to yield results favorable to the industry compared to studies where no financial ties to the industry existed.[29]

In terms of heart health and drugs, is it possible that it may not only be safer but also more effective simply to drink plenty of water? It's time to abandon the "high cholesterol" theory of heart disease. Consider what biochemist and nutritionist Udo Erasmus has said:

> Those whose income depends on treating diseases of our heart and arteries . . . who profit from the fact that sickness is better business than health, and whose priorities place profit before truth, cure, care, and life stand to lose much from a [dietary] solution to the puzzle of human cardiovascular disease. . . . In the end, cholesterol will be exonerated from its role as primary villain. . . . The accusing finger points at "experts" who concocted the cholesterol theory to drum up business by spreading fear.[30]

A FINAL NOTE ON EGGS

Those who raise chickens often describe them as intelligent creatures. If dogs or cats were kept in conditions like factory-raised chickens, the owners would be arrested for animal cruelty. Why do the owners of these unfortunate hens get away with this? Not only is it inhumane behavior, but it results in inferior-quality eggs. The typical supermarket egg is less than what it should be and may even contain traces of antibiotics and pesticides from the grains fed to the hens. Like powdered eggs, these are best avoided.

Chickens like space. They like to scratch and peck. The grasses, seeds, and insects they consume in a free-range environment contribute not only to larger amounts of the important fat-soluble vitamins A and D, but also to a larger amount of the omega-3 fatty acids—more heart-healthy nutrients that are lacking in most American diets.

From a humane standpoint, "cage-free" eggs are more desirable than factory-raised eggs, especially if their diet consists of organic feed. Better yet, of course, would be free-range eggs with their better fat profile. Also, it is now possible in some areas to purchase eggs from hens fed a special diet of algae or flax seeds, which greatly enhances levels of omega-3 fatty acids.

The omega-3s not only raise levels of HDL and decrease the risk of heart disease, they delay the loss of immunological function and inhibit the growth of breast and prostate cancer. Many Americans have absolutely no levels of omega-3 (EPA and DHA) in their blood tissues.[31] These new supplemented eggs boost the levels of DHA nearly fourfold so that three of these eggs have the omega-3 content of one fish meal. The eggs' supply of linolenic acid is increased thirtyfold. Our bodies have the capability of converting this acid into the other, healthy, omega-3 (EPA). Some chickens on a special diet also produce eggs with higher levels of vitamin E. Look for these as well as for the organic and free-range eggs.

In terms of eating eggs, it is best to cook the egg whites. Frequent consumption of raw egg whites can cause nutrient deficiencies. The whites contain a substance called avidin, which interferes with the absorption of biotin, an important B vitamin. Light cooking neutralizes avidin as well as other substances in raw egg whites (trypsin inhibitors), which interfere with the digestion of proteins.

Growing up as children we often heard the saying, "An apple a day keeps the doctor away." We certainly do not wish to demean apples; they are a wonderful food. But perhaps we should change that old saying to "An egg (or two) a day keeps the doctor away." This, it seems, would be good advice, particularly for those wishing to rebuild health. For those already experiencing robust health, it must be remembered that diversifying the food we eat helps to prevent developing allergies to specific foods. Though egg allergies are not common, it would be a shame to develop an allergy to eggs—a near-perfect food.

■■ TIPS: ■■

Good sources of the antioxidants lutein and zeaxanthin: eggs, broccoli, spinach.

Drinking plenty of water (five or more glasses a day) can protect the heart. Try replacing other drinks with pure, filtered or natural spring water flavored with a twist of lemon or lime.

To get the greatest benefit from eating eggs, purchase organic eggs from free-range chickens. They are higher in omega 3s; vitamins A, D, and E; and do not contain the potentially dangerous traces of antibiotics and pesticides that regular supermarket eggs do.

PLASTICS AND MICROWAVES

Propaganda: Plastics and microwaves save work and are more sanitary, which makes them healthier to use.

Reality: Hospitals and LaLeche Leagues now advise against microwaving human breast milk because it destroys immunological function. Science verifies that dangerous xenoestrogens and other chemicals leach into our food from plastic containers, especially when heated.

WHAT HAVE WE DONE TO OUR FOOD?

Scientists are alarmed. Certain animal species such as seal, otter, and mink are in decline. Many suffer from reproductive tract cancers. Bats and panthers are showing hormone dysfunction; fish and alligators are becoming feminized. Frogs and salamanders are turning up deformed. What's going on here? These problems are not so evident in humans. Or are they? Could there be ramifications for our species?

Many scientists think so. They are aware of the increasing rates of human breast and testicular cancers, and they also notice that sperm counts have greatly declined in the last forty years or so. (Does the tremendous popularity of Viagra indicate that men may be having serious hormonal problems?) A substantial number of researchers point a finger at environmental toxins like DDT and PCBs—those foreign estrogens, "xenoestrogens," which disrupt the endocrine system.[1]

Since the endocrine systems of all vertebrates use similar hormones to regulate development and reproduction, deformed fish should be seen as a warning sign for humans. The ground water and surface water in which the animals live are often contaminated with these estrogenic chemicals, which find their way into our food and water as well. Two rivers in England are so polluted with estrogens and estrogen-mimics downstream from sewage treatment plants that 100 percent of the fish have become feminized.[2] With falling human sperm counts, perhaps this type of pollution has become a bizarre way in which an overpopulated and heavily industrialized world begins to "decrease the excess population." Naturally, in the United States, chemical manufacturers usually deny the health link between xenoestrogens and human problems, saying nothing has been proven.

Studies linking DDT and PCBs to breast cancer, for example, have been mixed. Research showing higher levels of these chemicals in women with breast cancer have recently been countered by a Nurses Study that found no cause and effect. The problem here is that we don't know whether these particular xenoestrogens are a true problem when they accumulate in the later stages of a woman's life—or whether they do their damage by virtue of fetal exposure or even from exposure during puberty. It is unclear. What is also unclear is how the hundreds of xenoestrogens that have *not* been studied interact with one another.

ESTROGENS GALORE

Although these endocrine disrupters are very weak by comparison to natural hormones, the synergistic effect of several working together make their potency quite troublesome. And when you consider how many women and children who are not only exposed to DDT and PCBs but also are inclined to slather their skin with sunscreens that are notorious for containing estrogen-mimics, we appear to have a rather serious and complicated problem.

Some of these hormone disrupters like the pesticides DDT, DDD, lindane, and heptachlor have been banned in many countries including the United States. Some of them, however, are still manufactured in the United States or by U.S. corporations abroad, and then sold to developing countries for use on their crops. In 1994 the United States exported nine tons of these banned pesticides per day.[3] Some foreign crops treated with these chemicals come back to us so that we are consuming some of what we have banned. This *circle of poison* creates a worldwide problem.

Besides the "banned" pesticides, countless other xenoestrogens continue to be produced and used in the United States—two billion pounds of pesticides alone each year. Add to that the hormone disrupters leaching into the air, food, and water in the form of industrial waste, pharmaceuticals, and the hormones fed to livestock, and it is easy to see a possible reason why young girls are reaching puberty much earlier than they did a hundred years ago—or even twenty years ago. Heavy use of phytoestrogen-laden soy formula, of course, must not be left out of the equation.

The point of all this (in terms of nutrition) is that cancer and developmental problems associated with these chemicals may have evolved from another pathway into our food and water—the very packaging of the food we eat. The problem stems from some of our plastics.

PROBLEMS WITH SOFT PLASTIC

In order to make certain plastics more flexible, chemical plasticizers called "phthalates" (pronounced THAL-ates) are added to such items as tablecloths, blood bags, shower curtains, beer bottle caps, and PVC toys (rubber duckies). Phthalates are classified as cancer-causing substances.[4] Some products contain as much as 40 percent phthalates by weight. Millions of tons of these chemicals produced every year find uses in cosmetics, adhesives, inks, detergents, solvents, lubricants, paints, and vinyl flooring. The most common phthalate, DEHP, is used in the cap-sealing resins of bottled foods and in the heat-seal coatings on metal foils (as in yogurt). This, and other endocrine-disrupting phthalates also find their way into many baby foods and infant formulas. Significant amounts of DEHP migrate to foods like those in retail packed lunches. The source here is the disposable gloves used by the workers who put the lunches together. PVC gloves have a high percentage of DEHP.

Also of concern is another plasticizer, DEHA, found in at least one brand of PVC cling wrap sold for home use (Reynolds) and in a number of brands of plastic wrap used by supermarkets to seal fresh food products. Although apparently not a hormone mimic like its phthalate cousin DEHP, DEHA leaches into foods wrapped in such plastic in substantial amounts—especially into fat-containing foods like cheese and meat, which have a strong attraction for this substance. DEHA migrates into foods in even greater amounts when in contact with foods that are being microwaved. These amounts typically exceed limits that have been established by the European Union. The disease-causing potential of DEHA is still not clear. For now, the U.S. EPA labels it a "possible human carcinogen." To be safe, it would be wise to avoid purchasing wraps containing this plasticizer for home use. Also check with your market to make sure they are not using DEHA-containing cling wrap.

As far as children's toys are concerned, a number of countries have banned the use of phthalates found in the PVC used in toys for children under three years of age—such as teething rings and pacifiers. Not willing to ruffle the plasticized feathers of the chemical industry, the United States now requires only warnings.

PROBLEMS WITH HARD PLASTICS

Another potentially dangerous xenoestrogen is contaminating our food and water as well—bisphenol-A. Found not only in some of the tooth sealants typically used by dentists on young children, this endocrine disrupter can be found in the lining of many canned foods. Canned foods are usually heated during processing. This heat increases the amount of bisphenol-A that enters into the food inside the can. Some canned foods examined contained 80 parts per billion. This is many times more than the amount reported to stimulate estrogen receptors and cause breast cancer cells to proliferate in the lab.[5]

Bisphenol-A is also linked to weight gain. When combined with insulin in animal studies, it increases the number of fat cells as well as their storage capacity.[6] It appears this may be an environmental factor adding further to those lifestyle and dietary practices that predispose so many Americans to obesity.

Although these estrogen-mimics are much less potent than natural hormones that are quickly broken down and excreted by the body, xeno-estrogens stick around much, much longer while doing their dirty work as they accumulate in our body fat. Some researchers even link fybrocystic breast disease, endometriosis, and birth defects to these chemicals. In animal studies some of these endocrine disrupters are transferred not only to the fetus,[7] but also to the nursing infant through breast milk.[8] Exposure in the earliest years of life is also linked to mental impairment[9]—perhaps one more factor involved with the seemingly high rates of attention deficit disorder so prevalent today. The negative impact on the infant's thyroid due to fluoride and excessive amounts of phytoestrogens in soy formula—along with its high manganese content—is also being targeted as a culprit in the early onset of puberty and childhood behavioral and attention disorders.[10]

PLASTIC WATER

Bisphenol-A leaches out of bottles made of a plastic called polycarbonate. This hard plastic can be identified with the number 7 inside the recycling triangle on the bottom of the bottle. (Avoid the chemicals leaching from bottles with the recycling numbers 3 and 6 as well.) The bluish two, three, and five-gallon water bottles are often made of polycarbonate, as well as the clear feeding bottles for infants. This is of special concern for the developing baby who is consuming significant doses of this form of estrogen in formula or breast milk—particularly when the liquid is heated.

While speaking of heating, never microwave foods covered with, or contained in, plastic. As we know, the microwave process increases the migration of hormone disrupters into the food. This, however, may not be the only reason to be concerned about using your microwave oven.

ARE MICROWAVES SAFE?

The use of microwave technology for cooking began about 40 years ago. One would think that there should be countless studies attesting to the safety of eating foods cooked in this manner. Very few can be found. This is surprising. Very peculiar. There should be stacks of studies. But what we find largely is research that shows, for example, that microwave cooking may preserve nutrients in certain instances or deplete nutrients in others. We find studies about how the texture or taste of food is altered, or how long to cook various foods. There is even a scientific study on how microwave ovens cook yellow cake! But what about how the food is altered?

Although microwave cooking is not the same as food irradiation, does the microwave process, perhaps, create new and potentially dangerous by-products, much like irradiating food does? Does the high heat generated damage the health-giving essential fatty acids and make them harmful? We do know that direct exposure to microwaves damages the body. A damaged oven or leaky seal can result in you getting cooked as well as the food. Studies have certainly dealt with this issue, and it is therefore recommended to stand five to ten feet away from an operating oven. But, again, what about the food?

A 1988 study involving microwave-cooked pumpkin seeds suggests that potentially cancer-causing, free-radical formation can occur through the destruction of unsaturated fatty acids.[11] A 2001 study revealed that roasting peanuts in a microwave oven created "some undesirable and harmful products."[12] There are concerns that microwaving food blocks the ability of certain antioxidants to be protective.[13] Even microwaved water appears to be altered. Plants watered with microwaved water were shown to grow at half the rate compared to those watered with conventionally warmed water.[14] These studies are a good start. But where are the follow-up studies examining the effects on a broad range of foods and liquids? One would think red flags should have been raised.

FLAGS RAISED AND TORN DOWN

In the 1980s, two Swiss researchers wanted some answers. Denied a grant from the Swiss government to conduct studies related to the safety of eating microwaved foods, they took it upon themselves to do the research on their own.

They examined the blood of individuals who consumed microwaved food, comparing it to the blood of people who ate the same food prepared conventionally. They found negative changes in both the red and white blood cells of the microwaved-food eaters, as well as rapidly raised cholesterol levels with the consumption of microwaved vegetables. Since there is no cholesterol in vegetables, it appears that the body produced higher amounts of its own cholesterol in order to fight off some assault created by the consumption of the microwaved food. Cholesterol rises during times of acute stress and also when the body begins to undergo cancerous changes.

There was quite a stir when wind of the study reached the Swiss population. Many citizens were reported to have rushed to stores to return microwave ovens they had received as Christmas gifts. The Swiss authorities and the microwave manufacturers were not pleased. The researchers, Doctors Hans Hertel and Bernard Blanc, were taken to court and convicted in 1993 of interfering with commerce. A gag order was placed on them preventing them from publicly talking or writing about the dangers of microwave ovens. They were prohibited from expressing their scientific conclusions under threat of fine and imprisonment. Specifically, the two scientists were prevented from saying that "food prepared in microwave ovens is dangerous to health and may lead to pathological changes in the blood as also indicative for the beginning of a cancerous process."[15,16]

SOME CORROBORATION

At about the same time, other researchers were finding that milk formula and expressed human milk were damaged by microwave heating. Formula heated in this fashion resulted in potentially dangerous molecular changes; amino acids were altered and turned into substances that are toxic to the kidneys, liver, and nervous system.[17]

In the case of human milk, disease-fighting capabilities were damaged even at low microwave temperatures.[18] Today the La Leche League officially advises not to heat breast milk with a microwave oven, not only because the milk is heated unevenly, but also because immunological properties are lost. Suffice it to say, hospital maternity wards today do not use microwave ovens for heating milk or formula.

EARLIEST—AND FORGOTTEN—RESEARCH

Compared to the communist oppression in the former U.S.S.R., we are grateful for our intellectual freedoms. It is ironic, however, that our free-market and individual liberties may have exacted an unexpected price: diminished scientific integrity. Though much of the scientific research in Russia during the 1970s was geared toward their military intentions and needs, they were not so much constrained by an economy in which research was controlled or dictated by big business and by commercial profitability. Though we may not like hearing it, their scientists, though controlled by the state, were looking for answers without regard to protecting profits or swaying public opinion; they were in many cases, it appears, looking for the truth of the matter. Though lagging behind the United States in terms of applied science, the Soviets seemed more advanced in some areas of pure research.

Understanding how microwaves impact food is a case in point. According to U.S. researcher William Kopp, the Russians conducted extensive research concerning the effects of microwaves on food, as did the the Germans during WWII. According to Mr. Kopp, some of the findings of this early research involving food cooked with microwaves include:

- A well-known carcinogen developed in heated meats.
- Proteins were destabilized.
- Cancer-causing agents were found in treated milk and cereal grains.
- Microwaved food consumption created malfunctions in the digestive and lymphatic systems.
- Free radicals were formed.
- More human stomach and intestinal cancers were observed in those consuming microwaved foods.
- The bioavailability of many vital nutrients decreased.
- All foods studied were damaged in some way.[19]

As a result of these studies, and because direct contact with microwaves is so very dangerous, the Soviets were reported to have outlawed the use of all microwave apparatus in 1976.[20] However, the ban was lifted during the next decade when social restructuring in the U.S.S.R. began, which included a drift toward a market economy (Perestroika).

WHAT TO DO?

Where does that leave us? Can Mr. Kopp's assertions be corroborated? Has it been absolutely proven that microwaved food is dangerous to eat? No. Has it been proven that it is safe? No. There are far too many unanswered questions—perhaps questions that certain special interest groups do not want answered. Mr. Kopp's research from the 1970s confirm much of what recent research has uncovered. But for Mr. Kopp, the release of his information was so explosive that he found it necessary to change his name and disappear.[21]

It appears that microwave technology became entrenched in our culture too quickly. Its implementation spread to the public segment and took hold before conclusive research could justify its use. It's too difficult now to stuff the genie back in the bottle.

There seems to be little incentive for research funds to be spent in this area. Business interests are too heavily invested in microwave technology.

And some researchers may be dissuaded from pursuing their own projects after learning about the threats and prosecution endured by Mr. Kopp and the Swiss scientists. However, there is at least one happy ending: In 1998 it was found that Dr. Hertel's right to free expression had been violated by the Swiss courts. The gag order was lifted and the doctor can now speak freely about his microwave research. He received a nice monetary award as well.

With so many health-related topics, there is always the risk-vs.-benefit assessment to be made. With regard to the endocrine disrupters found in some plastics, which are new to the human species: Until we know a lot more about how the fetus, infant, child, and adult are impacted by these substances, it makes sense to avoid them when we make food choices. Choose organic foods. Avoid liquids and foods stored and packaged in questionable plastics. This is not too difficult. We are already getting too many of these xenoestrogens from car exhaust, solvents, adhesives, vinyl products, sunscreens, and other sources. Until we have more research on how microwave ovens impact the food we eat, is the convenience of using one of them worth the possible risks? In terms of the health of infants, hospitals don't think so. Should we treat our own health with any less regard?

■■ TIPS: ■■

Go back to conventional cooking methods like the stovetop! Avoid purchasing plastic wraps for home use that are made with DEHA plasticizer—Reynolds Wrap is one of them. Check with your store to see if they are using DEHA-containing plastic to wrap deli foods.

Never microwave foods in plastic! This is especially important for the developing infant or child.

VITAMIN C

Propaganda: Vitamin C is totally safe and the higher the dose the better.

Reality: Megadoses may create nutritional imbalances.

TOO MUCH OF A GOOD THING?

"If a little is good, then more must be better" has become an American credo, especially in the field of health. The more soy the better, the more carbohydrates the better, and now, the more protein the better. What ever happened to balance and common sense?

The superstar of vitamins must surely be vitamin C (ascorbic acid). We are well aware of the benefits of this nutrient, how it protects against free-radical damage responsible for a host of diseases, how it strengthens blood vessels and collagen, how it strengthens the immune system, and how it's useful for just about any condition from asthma to vitiligo.

Such a well-researched vitamin certainly deserves the attention and praise it has garnered. It appears to be nontoxic in high doses, leading some scientists to suggest taking as many grams of the stuff as you can—up until you finally get diarrhea, a message from the body saying "enough already."

One of the reasons given for recommending huge doses of vitamin C comes from the study of animals. Almost all animals synthesize their own supplies of this vitamin. We humans don't. We rely solely on diet for our supply. But to match the amount of ascorbic acid produced by other animals we would need to consume megadoses of it in supplemental form. It would be impossible by diet alone to get enough vitamin C to match what the animals produce.

But haven't researchers noticed that we are different from the other animals? Maybe we don't need as much vitamin C, and that's why we evolved to obtain it from food sources.

HOW MUCH IS TOO MUCH?

The folks at the National Institutes of Health, as well as those at the National Academy of Sciences, have recommended a daily intake of just 200 mg, although up to 500 mg has been shown to be useful.[1] More than that is generally not used or absorbed efficiently by the body. In amounts over 500 mg you are rapidly flushing vitamin dollars down the toilet, it is implied.[2,3] This common-sense approach, however, is not accepted by the general public and by many researchers who suggest up to 50 times the recommended amount. After all, it's nontoxic.

In 1998 scientists in England created quite a stir when they suggested that doses over 500 mg a day could cause ascorbic acid to become a *pro*-oxidant instead of an *anti*-oxidant.[4] What this means is that, at high doses, our favorite vitamin creates free-radicals that could result in heart disease, cancer, and arthritis. These researchers were generally ridiculed in the press by some not willing to look deeper into the issue. How could a nontoxic substance create DNA damage? The public was told by supporters of the vitamin that the research in England was probably a fluke or just poorly designed. What is shown in a test tube must surely be different from what happens inside the human body. No need to stop gobbling the vitamin C pills, we were reassured by many.

However, the lead researcher of a more recent study at the University of Southern California suggested that vitamin supplements should not be substituted for a healthy, balanced diet. He had found that subjects consuming more than 500 mg of vitamin C developed greater wall thickness in the neck arteries, a sign of developing atherosclerosis.[5] Not a good sign at all. Again, the research was attacked. Something must be wrong with the study or methods, we were warned. Rather than simply say that we need to conduct more studies on the matter, some scientists could only attack. Apparently, it is oftentimes human nature to initially reject anything that counters our long-held beliefs. We don't want to hear that perhaps we were wrong about recommending megadoses of a "harmless" substance. Pride is often at stake. Admittedly, the recent research showing possible damage from excess vitamin C is not complete.

A 2002 study, however, seems to back the earlier USC study. Postmenopausal women with some coronary artery damage were given either hormone replacement therapy or daily supplementation with 1000 mg of vitamin C (along with 800 mg of vitamin E). There were more deaths in the HRT group as well as in the vitamin-supplemented group when compared to the control group. There was also a greater narrowing of the arteries. The researchers, therefore, found no benefit from treating such patients with either HRT or with vitamins C and E. "Instead, a potential for harm was suggested with each treatment."[6] Certainly, we need to know more, and we are finding out more. But in the meantime, caution is needed.

What has been forgotten by many is the fact that a nutrient doesn't have to be toxic in order to be dangerous in large amounts. Too much water can kill. What about vitamin C? Even beyond the possibility that it may become dangerously oxidative in moderately large amounts— amounts commonly taken by many adults in pill form—there is still another reason why too much C could be dangerous. And it has to do with balance.

A Delicate Balance

What does a "balanced diet" mean? It means getting nutrients in a way in which they optimally support one another. Through food, humans evolved to consume a myriad of vitamins and minerals, including ascorbic acid, which complement one another in the correct proportion. Since it takes some work to consume more than 500 mg of vitamin C a day in food we eat, what happens when we get more than that through supplementation?

Balance is thrown off, particularly with regard to iron and copper. Both metals, of course, are useful, but unlike vitamin C (perhaps) they are toxic in large amounts. And vitamin C regulates how much of these metals we absorb.

Although there are still many in this country who suffer from an iron deficiency that causes anemia, it is believed by many health experts that a large portion of the population is overconsuming iron, which pervades fortified cereals and multivitamin tablets. Cast-iron cookware contributes a fair amount of iron to the diet as do, surprisingly, stainless steel pots and pans.

Too much iron creates free radicals that lead to a risk of heart disease, accelerated aging, and cancer.[7] Excess iron may, as some researchers put it, "bestow immortality upon the cancer cell."[8] Also, some researchers suspect high levels of iron in the brain to be implicated in the development of Parkinson's disease.[9] Others have linked it to diabetes and to a dysfunctional immune system.[10]

If we are already getting too much iron, what happens when we toss down a couple of vitamin C pills with our meal? Absorption increases. Generally, the body has a mechanism to restrict the absorption of iron to about 10 percent, but in the presence of ascorbic acid, the absorption rate can increase by a factor of four.[11] This is not good news unless you are quite iron deficient.

Iron In and Copper Out

There is some evidence that large amounts of vitamin C in supplemental form convert iron in the body to a more dangerous form of iron, one that creates free radicals capable of mounting an attack on body parts, particularly the joints.[12] Vitamin C from food (as ascorbate) apparently is incapable of doing this, presumably because vitamin C in food works synergistically with many other antioxidants. Ascorbic acid in pill form, it must be remembered, is not the only form of vitamin C on the block.

Vitamin C in large amounts can kill certain cells.[13] This is thought to be of value when we need to destroy existing cancer cells. But what if we don't have cancer? Will it help as a cancer preventive? Apparently not.[14,15] What then will excess ascorbic acid do? First of all, in small amounts vitamin C needs to become an oxidant rather than an antioxidant. This is how it passes the blood-brain barrier to get to our brain tissue where it becomes a valuable antioxidant once again.[16] But what happens if we have too much C, especially in combination with iron? Apparently, greater oxidization occurs, creating billions of free radicals that can damage DNA,[17] with little evidence that it can decrease oxidative damage to DNA, except in those greatly lacking in this nutrient.[18,19] Additional research seems to back up what the besieged British scientists have found;[20,21] ascorbic acid might be involved in promoting cancer by virtue of the DNA damage it causes, with or without the presence of iron.[22]

Further bad news (sorry) involves human studies in which extra vitamin C becomes particularly *pro*-oxidative—leading to tissue damage—when the body is already subject to inflammatory conditions (arthritis, cardiovascular disease, muscle injury, Alzheimer's disease, etc.).[23] Under these circumstances, more dangerous iron is released. These findings led to a recommendation by the lead researcher to limit vitamin C to no more than 100 mg when inflammation is present.

MORE HEAVY METAL

Vitamin C's action on copper, however, is the exact opposite of what it does to iron. Ascorbic acid depletes copper, a mineral that, according to the USDA, most Americans are deficient in. Copper, with high concentrations in the brain, helps to regulate blood cholesterol and protect against high blood pressure. In the proper amounts copper also helps with free-radical scavenging and aids in bone development. Too much vitamin C can prevent us from getting enough of this important mineral.[24,25]

Perhaps this is one reason we have evolved into a species that derives its C from food only—to ensure that we do not synthesize so much of it that it reduces copper to levels so low that brain development and intelligence are hampered. Low copper levels can create brain dysfunctions.[26,27]

Those zinc tablets many Americans are now consuming in excess may contribute to the further decline of copper in the body.[28,29] And to make matters worse, it now seems that the extra iron we are getting, thanks in part to vitamin C, may further inhibit copper bioavailability.[30] Anyone consuming sugar? More bad news for copper.[31]

If most of us are already low in copper, and many of us already have adequate or dangerously high amounts of iron, it appears almost foolish to upset the balance of these minerals with large amounts of vitamin C.

Help or Hinder Arthritis?

Further speculation on the overdosing of ascorbic acid leads to the subject of hyaluronic acid. This substance can be found in all cells of the body, with the highest concentration in connective tissue, eyes, cartilage, synovial fluid, and skin. It's hydrating effect on skin makes it something of an antiaging substance. It's lubricating properties in the joints help protect against arthritis. The ever-so-popular glucosamine sulfate helps to stimulate production of this important component of synovial fluid. Arthritic joints are deficient in this substance, which is sometimes injected by physicians into the joints of patients to restore flexibility and to reduce pain.

In Japan, 10 percent of the villagers of Yuzuri Hara are over 85 years old. This is ten times the norm in America. They rarely need a doctor and most are free of the diseases that plague Western cultures. Their skin sometimes shows no sign of aging. It is speculated that their diet, which consists of certain sweet potatoes and roots, stimulates the production of hyaluronic acid.[32] Sadly, many of their children who have adopted a more Western diet are dying before their parents, leading to speculation that a reduced intake of hyaluronic acid may be one of the factors involved.

Connection to Vitamin C

Researchers in this country are now looking into the use of hyaluronic acid to stop the progression of emphysema. It's a valuable substance in the body that can aid in wound repair and modulate the inflammatory process. But it can be degraded by ascorbic acid.[33]

Although normal amounts of vitamin C seem joint-protective, a high level of this vitamin (which brings joint-destructive iron with it) seems to override the body's protection against the degradation of hyaluronic acid. For the tissue, this means less ability to hold on to water. For the joints, this means they become more vulnerable to attacks by free radicals with less capacity to stay lubricated. This surely must be one of the signs of accelerated aging. For menopausal women faced with the reality of rapidly aging skin, the main culprit appears to be a lack of estrogen which, before the decline, supported the production of hyaluronic acid to maintain healthy skin.[34]

Could excess vitamin C be an accomplice to all this mayhem? To be fair, it's unclear to what extent ascorbic acid degrades hyaluronic acid in the human body, but if the researchers in England are correct about any amount of vitamin C over 500 mg becoming oxidative, the prospect of keeping joints, eyes, and skin healthy with megadoses of C becomes quite unlikely. Even dangerous perhaps.

Are we "fooling with Mother Nature" when we upset the balance of nutrients with more vitamin C than the body was designed for? Is it an evolutionary "mistake" that we can obtain ascorbic acid only from food? Animals that generate their own C send it to the liver where it is converted to various more useful mineral ascorbates. When we obtain vitamin C from food sources, we are also ingesting these valuable ascorbates which work in conjunction with ascorbic acid.

A CAUTION

We are well-advised to take note of Finnish and U.S. research in which it was found that smokers given the supplemental vitamin A precursor, beta carotene, increased their chances of getting cancer.[35] In another major study—involving those not necessarily smokers—supplemental beta carotene proved to be of no value at all.[36] Further research has suggested that the *pro*-oxidative effects of supplemental vitamin A or beta carotene is capable of damaging DNA and could lead to cancer.[37]

We could surmise that beta carotene alone may create a deficiency in the other many carotenoids found in food, some of which may offer greater anticancer benefits than what beta carotene has been thought to offer. It should be remembered that an excess of vitamin A has been shown to lead to higher rates of bone fracture, presumably when it is not balanced with enough vitamin D. A researcher in vitamin A studies has claimed that we need "a rethinking of the use of natural compounds as chemoprevention agents. These agents should no longer be regarded as harmless, but as having potential toxicities."[38] *Mega-supplements* may be creating *mega-imbalances*.

It appears that vitamin C may fall into this category. However, didn't Linus Pauling himself recommend megadoses of vitamin C? Yes, he personally consumed 15,000–18,000 mg per day. But what does his official organization currently have to say about the matter? Professor Balz Frei, a nutrition expert at the Linus Pauling Institute notes that, although someone in a diseased state may benefit from large quantities of vitamin C, there is not enough evidence to say that healthy people would benefit at all from vitamin C supplementation. He says: "The Linus Pauling

Institute does not endorse megadoses. Our advice is to eat a healthy diet rich in fruits and vegetables."[39] A breath of fresh air.

Unless vitamin C is to be used like a drug in treating illness—or unless this vitamin is depleted by a high consumption of sugar or by excessive sun exposure—or by cigarettes, alcohol, caffeine, heavy metal intoxication, aspirin, birth control pills, and perhaps stress, 200 mg a day would be wise. This is the amount recommended by the Pauling Institute, contrary to popular belief. Otherwise, up to 500 mg per day might be a good idea depending upon a person's lifestyle or surfeit of bad habits that quickly deplete stores of this nutrient.

Vitamin C from food, of course, is best. But if you are adverse to citrus fruits, strawberries, cantaloupe, kiwi, broccoli, tomatoes, cabbage, peppers, potatoes, and lettuce, a small supplement could be considered. Avoid plain ascorbic acid because it can adversely affect the delicate alkaline/acid balance in the body. Mineral ascorbates, like calcium ascorbate, are a good choice. Be cautious about balance.

▪▪ Tips: ▪▪

200–500 mg as a daily intake has been shown to be useful.

Cigarettes, alcohol, caffeine, heavy-metal toxicity, aspirin, birth control pills, stress, sugar, and excess sun exposure deplete vitamin C in the body, in which case supplementation may be recommended.

Whole food sources for balanced vitamin C are: citrus fruits, strawberries, cantaloupe, kiwi, broccoli, cabbage, tomatoes, peppers, potatoes, and lettuce.

FOOD IRRADIATION

Propaganda: Irradiating our food increases valuable shelf life and protects us from foodborne *E. coli*.

Reality: There have been almost no comprehensive studies on the safety of irradiated food, and it is proven that irradiation of food increases the potent cancer-causing mold aflatoxin, depletes nutrients, and may make the body more susceptible to cancer and other illness.

THE PUBLIC AS GUINEA PIGS

During a three-year period, six million Americans placed a call to Miss Cleo's psychic hot line for advice on love and money. Do we need more evidence than this that the general public is rather gullible and therefore easy prey to scams and unsound advice? Perhaps many Americans slept through their high school science classes.

With an audience of ten million radio listeners, "America's Doctor," Dean Edell, serves as an antidote to our nation's broad irrationality. He should be commended for his attempt to integrate reason, common sense, and a scientific approach into a healthy lifestyle. He states, "The truth is too important when it comes to your health." Bravo. But you have to scratch your head when you read what he has to say about food irradiation: "Irradiation doesn't cause cancer-causing substances or reduce nutritional value . . . I see nothing wrong with irradiating (food) to make it safer to eat."[1] On what science is this statement based? On what evidence?

Writing for the *Bulletin of the Atomic Scientists* is Dr. Donald B. Louria, Chairman of the Preventative Medicine Department at the New Jersey Medical School in Newark, N.J.: "The FDA judged safety (of irradiation) based on five of 441 available toxicity studies. Of the available literature, claimed the FDA, only these five animal studies were 'properly conducted, fully adequate by 1980 toxicological standards and able to stand alone in support of safety.'"

But when these studies were reviewed at the Department of Preventive Medicine and Community Health of the New Jersey Medical School, two were found to be methodologically flawed, either by poor statistical analyses or because negative data were disregarded. One of the two also suggested that irradiated food could have adverse effects on older animals. In a third FDA–cited study, animals fed a diet of irradiated food experienced weight loss and miscarriage, almost certainly due to irradiation-induced vitamin E dietary deficiency. This study, which used foods that had been subjected to large doses of radiation, indicated that irradiated food suffered nutritional loss. These three studies do not document the safety of food irradiation, and why the FDA relied on them is mystifying.[2]

BAD SCIENCE

The other two studies used by the FDA to approve food irradiation, although sound, involved the use of radiation below that which is currently approved. Good science dictates that new studies be done based on the much higher radiation used on food. Instead, the FDA has now relied on old research it had earlier "failed to include as methodologically sound." (Louria)

It appears that the public at large is being subjected to a large scientific experiment. For ethical reasons, in the United States it is difficult to prove the safety of irradiated food on human test subjects. In China and India, however, where ethical considerations are minimized, human test subjects eating irradiated food developed chromosomal abnormalities.[3,4] Subsequent research has tried to downplay these serious findings,[5] but even in doing so, the researchers admitted that, in the case of irradiating wheat, the fatty acid content is altered. Toxic peroxides are created.[6] These substances can lead to cancer and heart disease and also suppress liver and immune function.[7]

A further problem is not that the food contains leftover radiation, but rather that it contains something called "unique radiolytic products," not to mention well-known cancer-causing agents like formaldehyde and benzene. According to Public Citizen: "These products (URPs) are free radicals, which set off chain reactions in the body that destroy antioxidants, tear apart cell membranes, and make the body more susceptible to cancer, diabetes, heart disease, liver damage, muscular breakdown, and other serious health problems."[8]

One recently discovered class of URPs (cyclobutanones)—substances not found in nature—also turn up in irradiated food. They have been ignored by the FDA even though they have been implicated in colon cancer[9] and have been found to "cause genetic damage in rats, and genetic and cellular damage in human and rat cells."[10] Some experts believe children to be especially vulnerable to these untested substances.[11]

NUKE THOSE CRITTERS

Simply put, irradiated food doesn't glow in the dark, but it contains many substances whose properties are unclear. Some of them have been tested in the lab and are suspected of being carcinogenic because they may cause mutations. Irradiated food fed to lab animals has resulted in chromosomal damage, vitamin K and E deficiencies, internal bleeding, increases in embryonal deaths, nutritional muscular dystrophy, decreases in newborn survival rates, and mutations.[12]

According to John Gofman, M.D., Ph.D., Professor Emeritus of Molecular and Cell Biology at the University of California, Berkeley, "Our ignorance about these foreign compounds (radiolytic products) makes it simply a fraud to tell the public that 'we know' irradiated food would be safe to eat."[13] And despite what we are frequently told by health authorities, there is plenty of evidence that treated food loses vitamin content, especially vitamins A, C, E, and members of the B complex.[14,15] Cooking irradiated food appears to accentuate the nutrient loss.[16]

Touted as a way to extend food shelf-life and to eliminate food-borne pathogens like *E. coli* and salmonella, what promoters don't mention is the fact that irradiation actually increases in a huge way the amount of a very potent cancer-causing mold (aflatoxin).[17] It is also conceivable that irradiation could spawn mutant forms of certain harmful micro-organisms. (This would make a good movie.) Promoters of irradiation cite the need to eliminate these dangerous bacteria from the food supply, but widespread use of this technology is likely to allow meat processors to become even more unsanitary in their practices. We have safer and more effective sanitation methods available.[18]

By simply increasing the number of Department of Agriculture tests for pathogens in meat and poultry during the last two years (2001–2003), levels of salmonella have dropped significantly. But instead of cracking down on careless food processors or beefing up food inspections—and instead of promoting other existing technologies to kill harmful pathogens—the U.S. government has opted to benefit industry and, at the same time, play a game of chance with public health.

ARSENIC—A SIDEBAR

As proof of the regrettable way in which government agencies regard public health, we need not look further than the issue of arsenic in drinking water. After years of study, years of debate, and years of delay, under the Clinton administration the limit of cancer-causing arsenic allowed in public water systems was to be dropped from 50 parts per billion to 10 ppb. At first the Bush administration had some reservations about upholding this new limit, but under pressure relented. The new limit will be enforced. But why 10 ppb?

Even at 3 ppb arsenic in water creates a high cancer risk. Many scientists and health organizations, however, recommend a maximum contaminant level for arsenic to be set at 3 ppb, not 10 ppb, which is estimated to result in 1 fatal cancer death for every 10,000 people. The EPA's normal risk standard for chemical exposure is 1 in 1,000,000.

But some experts expect that 1 in 1,000 persons who drink water contaminated even at the 3-ppb level could develop lung or bladder cancer, according to Dr. Robert Goyer, who chaired the National Research Council committee that reviewed arsenic risks.[19] To reach the new standard, the EPA estimates that the cost to filter the water for most people would be less than three dollars per month.[20] This amount would be higher for some very small water systems (for which federal subsidies would likely be available). Even so, many groups have complained about lowering the acceptable limit for arsenic because of these higher costs, low as they seem.

THREE DOLLARS MUST BE WHAT THE MARKET CAN BEAR

So the limit has been set at 10 ppb for the simple reason of cost. It is interesting to note what EPA Chief Christine Whitman had to say about setting this new standard: "... a standard of 10 ppb protects public health based on the best available science and ensures that the cost of the standard is achievable."[21] Well, 10 ppb is not based on the best science and does not protect the public very well at all. Many citizens will suffer from the terrible effects of arsenic in their water at that level: nervous system disorders, heart problems, and the cancers of the prostate, skin, kidney, liver, bladder and lung. What the 10-ppb level does is save money. It is much cheaper not to remove so much of the stuff. The lives of American citizens have been reduced to a dollar amount.

Here's a suggestion: Since the toxic fluoride chemicals (silicofluorides) currently being added to the water of over half of the American population contain measurable amounts of arsenic, why don't we first stop adding arsenic to the water before deciding how much to remove? The dollars saved by not having to pay to fluoridate public water systems could then be applied to removing the rest of the arsenic to levels below 3 ppb. Does this make too much sense?

BACK TO THE FOOD

What does all this have to do with food irradiation? The arsenic issue illustrates the government's lack of regard for public health and highlights its high regard for black numbers in the ledger. In short, it should be no surprise then that the government is going to save lots of bucks by convincing the public to accept food irradiation. There is a lot of radioactive waste out there. It's expensive to keep and to store safely. So if the Department of Energy can spread radioactive cobalt-60 and cesium-137 throughout the country in hundreds of food processing plants, they would be tickled pink. Yet have they considered the hazards involved with shipping it, preventing accidents at the plants, and making sure this dangerous material is protected from terrorist threat?

Dr. Louria provides another possible reason for our government's interest in food irradiation:

> Some critics charge that the Energy Department has been even more devious. They claim that the department was less interested in disposing of cesium than it was in overturning the ban on reprocessing civilian nuclear fuel. These critics claim that the department calculated that widespread food irradiation would eventually deplete the available supplies of cesium 137. At that point, the irradiation industry would begin to lobby for the reprocessing of spent fuel, and the department could use the industry to overcome the political and economic obstacles to reprocessing nuclear fuel. Once reprocessing was permitted, the Energy Department could separate the plutonium in spent fuel, which it could then use in weapons.[22,23]

This may sound exceedingly cynical. How could anyone be so deceitful and risk endangering public health and safety? Well, here's a concrete example of deceit: Some irradiating food processors are now advertising to the public that what they do to food is "cold pasteurization" or "electronic pasteurization." They use these euphemisms to mislead the public. They don't use the the the term "irradiation." They know that some people suspect that the treated food is "radioactive" and are frightened about irradiated food—for *good* reason—even if not for the *right* reason.

IS YOUR FOOD IRRADIATED?

Fortunately, our eggs, fruit, vegetables, meats, and so on must be labeled if they have been irradiated. Unfortunately, packaged foods that contain irradiated items do not have to show the "radura" symbol. Nor do restaurants. And as far as the National School Lunch Program is concerned—a program in which the USDA has forbidden the use of irradiation, the Bush Administration has proposed making a change in this policy. It has planned to drop expensive salmonella testing, which was required during the Clinton Administration, in favor of irradiating the beef that is served in school lunches. A recently passed bill has given the USDA the authority to proceed, and this government agency has just announced its intentions to do so.

"The government's assertion that irradiated food is safe for human consumption does not even pass the laugh test," says Samuel S. Epstein, M.D., Emeritus professor of environmental and occupational medicine at University of Illinois School of Public Health, Chicago. "Exposing America's school children to the hazards of irradiated food is reckless negligence, compounded by the absence of any warning to parents."[24]

Industry, however, is quite happy about this development. It is reported that during the year 2000, food companies and industry groups with a major stake in the proliferation of irradiated food gave $3.3 million to national Republican Party committees and federal candidates and $654,000 to the Democrats.[25]

Again, it's about money—and once again our health is at risk This gives us another good reason to eat whole, unprocessed, organic foods as much as possible. Know what you eat. And please, give Dr. Dean Edell a call.

■■ TIPS: ■■

Avoid foods marked with the Radura symbol. Packaged foods are not required to carry this symbol, so check with your store. Also, restaurants are not required to indicate whether the food they serve is irradiated or not.

Food-industry marketers are now using the term "cold pasteurization" or "electronic pasteurization" instead of "irradiated."

VEGETARIANISM

Propaganda: Vegetarians are healthier. If you want to be healthy, eat less meat.

Reality: Many vegetarians fall for all of the food industry's confusing, fallacious propaganda by avoiding meat while consuming high amounts of low-quality carbohydrates, highly processed and chemical-laden foods, and unfermented soy. This can lead to serious health problems.

ETHICAL AND DIETARY CONSIDERATIONS

There is little question that humans are designed to eat meat. We are omnivores. Our paleolithic ancestors thrived on the wild game that made up a large part of their diet. Traditional cultures from around the world have all consumed animal products in one degree or another for robust health.[1]

And yet, it is possible for some folks to maintain health on a vegetarian diet—particularly if it allows for dairy and eggs. Some individuals are genetically suited to a meatless diet, but in the United States they appear to be in the minority. Even fewer can attain optimal health on a strict vegetarian (vegan) regimen. Those who reject all animal foods like eggs, dairy, and honey often choose this lifestyle as a means of making a political or moral statement. Though we are omnivores, they rightly claim that we don't have to eat animal foods. Many vegans also avoid clothing from animal sources like furs, leather, and silk, and refuse to buy anything made with animal by-products (certain cosmetics, for example). Presumably vegans, to be consistent, do not drive cars or ride bicycles in order to avoid animal substances found in brake fluid and in tires.

A lifestyle based on such high principles deserves respect. Any proper moral system must have as its top priority the elimination or prevention of human suffering. Those who choose a vegetarian lifestyle for spiritual or moral reasons, as opposed to purely health considerations, often extend their sense of compassion to the animal kingdom. They are saddened by the conditions in which factory-farmed animals are raised. An overcrowded, unsanitary environment where animals are treated like objects instead of sentient beings should outrage us all. Profit at the expense of the well-being of the animals should not be tolerated. Vegetarians are correct to cease their financial support of an inhumane food industry.

Would the vegetarians, however, consider consuming meat and eggs from animals raised and treated properly—with care and respect—as exemplified by the common multipurpose farm of the past or by the love shown to animals by countless young "future farmers of America"?

Would meat-eating become an option when animals are allowed to free-range, to fully express their animality in a caring environment? In exchange for their good care they would then be given the opportunity to return the favor by serving a noble cause—that of giving themselves up to feed and nurture us. Would this matter? Perhaps not.

SOME PHILOSOPHY

We would hope that vegetarians have weighed these thoughts and have also considered the following: Ancient and traditional societies often had a more holistic view of the world. Life was One. All life was sacred. When animals were eaten, it was often done with gratitude and reverence. One extremely healthy African tribe, the Neurs, regarded the liver as the seat of the soul. To nourish their soul they felt it important to consume the liver of animals. Thus, the liver was a source of power. It was regarded as particularly sacred, and they would touch it only with tools—not the hands.[2] The value of the animal and its role in providing health was not undervalued.

In many ways modern society has lost sight of the interconnectness of all things. Shelling out only a buck for a burger keeps us removed from our food's source. In this country such food is too cheap, due in part to government subsidies, and it's too easily obtained. Food no longer sustains; it titillates us instead. We have lost reverence for many things, especially food. Appreciation for the rich web, the complex tapestry of life, has given way to a sense of dualism in which we no longer have a direct connection to the natural world. The ego is separated from everything else, and it has become difficult to see how we, as intelligent animals, exist as one of the threads of the fabric of the universe. We no longer see the whole. We divide, categorize, and prioritize all that is around us.

We do this with living creatures as well. We may squash the spider, but refuse to eat the fish. We drive our vehicles, which splatter countless creatures on the windshield or crush them under the wheels, but we refuse to eat an egg or have a taste of honey out of concern that some bees were harmed in the honey-collecting process. The point is: In a spiritual world view that holds that there is nothing but soul, and in a world view where even in the inanimate realm there is nothing but consciousness, it makes little sense to avoid the butter and the meat and, instead, yank out the vegetables by the roots (ouch!). There is nothing but life. It is artificial at best to confer a higher status to the chicken than to the turnip. The distinction made between plant and animal life is the very "trap" that may ensnare those who follow the vegan doctrine, according to American Zen Master (and Buddhist ethicist) Robert Aitken: "It is not possible to evade the natural order of things: everything in the universe is in symbiosis with every other thing. . . . Doctrines, including Buddhism, are meant to be used. Beware of them taking life of their own, for then they use us."[3]

Our anthropomorphic attitudes prevent us from seeing that the animal may be no more sentient or suffer no more than the plant. Peter Tompkins and Christopher Bird note in their wonderful book *The Secret Life of Plants*: "Evidence now supports the vision of the poet and the philosopher that plants are living, breathing, communicating creatures, endowed with personality and the attributes of soul. It is only we, in our blindness, who have insisted on considering them automata."[4]

SELF-SACRIFICE

Even after considering these arguments, those who thoughtfully elect to maintain vegetarian habits deserve praise for their particular moral course of action, if not for their selflessness. For it is reasonable to suggest that many vegetarians (vegans especially) may be sacrificing their own welfare (health) for the life of the animals. According to some religious thought, suffering is inextricably woven into the fabric of existence. Though we may wince to see the lion kill and devour the antelope, we can't stop the lion from doing what makes sense in the entire scheme of things. To what extent can or should we deny our own nature? Most vegetarians wish to reduce suffering, but if their own suffering (ill-health) is caused by an inadequate diet—a diet without animal products—then, ultimately, little has been gained, particularly if a lack of energy and a lack of robust health compromises their ability to do other good works in the world. Author and teacher Charles Eisenstein believes that "the moral question to ask oneself about food is not 'Was there killing?' but rather, 'Is this food taken in rightness and harmony?' "[5]

What about those who choose to be vegetarians solely for health considerations, thinking that they will attain better health by avoiding meat? As mentioned, it is possible to be a healthy vegetarian if one has the suitable biochemistry and genetic makeup. But it is very difficult and very risky for the rest of us. Nutritionists have hundreds of stories involving clients coming into the office with health problems that are reversed by adding animal fat and protein to the diet.

Many of these clients had felt good at first on a vegetarian diet. The high fiber, fruits, and vegetables may have initiated a cleansing process that counteracted years of a typical, unhealthy American diet replete with junk food and harmful, processed meats and fats. Followers of low-fat or no-fat vegetarian programs often have great initial success. They feel healthier and more energized. But as time goes by, those not extremely careful in their vegetarian food choices begin to show the effects of a lack of protein and a lack of many important nutrients, especially the important fats like the omega-3s. They come to the nutritionist with skin and hair dryness, menstrual irregularities, loss of energy, blood-sugar problems, sleep disorders, and even weight gain despite an overall decrease of caloric consumption.

To those with the biological capacity to maintain health and energy on a vegetarian diet, we tip our hats. We are grateful to have such people among us; they tread more lightly on this planet. For those struggling with health on such a diet, and for those whose refusal to consume animal foods makes eating a chore and adds daily stress to life due to food cravings left unsatisfied, it may be time to reconsider. Perhaps it's time to participate more fully in all the food choices available—to enjoy eating once more instead of fearing it. We can once again eat with joy—a joy that is imbued with a sense of reverence and gratitude. It's time, therefore, to take a look at some of the potential pitfalls of a vegetarian diet.

THE RESEARCH STUDIES

Some readers may be thinking that there can't be that many problems that are not easily remedied by tweaking the vegetarian diet here and there. After all, don't studies show that vegetarian populations show better health in general? Doesn't the research indicate that they generally have less heart disease, lower blood pressure, less prostate cancer, etc.? Some, but not all, studies show this to be so. Some research, however, indicates that the opposite is true, as in the case of heart disease.[6,7] Some studies, when reexamined, show that there is little difference in certain disease rates between the two groups. When evaluating the diet–disease connection, it must be remembered that vegetarians in general are more health-conscious to begin with and take better care of themselves—less smoking and alcohol consumption, for example. A viable study must take this into account.

Good research should also consider to what extent nonvegetarians consume chemical-laden, disease-causing processed meats. Are the meat-eaters consuming hormone-free, free-range beef and eggs? Or are vegetarian groups being compared to the general junk and fast-food-eating populations? We must also remember the findings of Dr. Weston Price who found the healthiest cultures eating substantial amounts of either fish, meat, or raw dairy foods. They did not show evidence of the kind of diseases attributed to the nonvegetarians of today. It has long been assumed from studies that meat-eaters had a greater incidence of colon cancer than vegetarians. When the research was looked at more carefully, it was found that the type of meat made a difference. Fresh, unadulterated meat was not connected to colon cancer; "lunch meats," hot dogs, and the like were implicated. In addition, colon cancer is related to high intakes of the omega-6 and hydrogenated oils.[8]

FOOD AND LONGEVITY

It must be noted that there are some vegetarians who also eat terrible foods as well. As long as what they consume has no fat, they sometimes feel comfortable eating huge amounts of nutrient-poor, refined carbohydrates and other sugary foods. As long as it's not meat then they think it's all right. These folks are probably no better off than their fast-food burger-eating counterparts. Can we compare these vegetarians to the average populace? You see, it is difficult to draw firm conclusions one way or another from many of these studies until we know more specific details about the quality of the food consumed when we attempt to assess rates of a particular disease.

The more useful study, perhaps, would be one that is more inclusive and that accounts for all life-threatening diseases—a longevity study. Do vegetarians outlive the meat eaters? Again, the results are mixed. Some studies say yes, and others point to a reduced life-span for the vegetarians, particularly for the women.[9]

If we look at the rates of heart disease in vegetarians, a number of studies indicate that there is less ischemic heart disease in the nonmeat-eaters. But then how do we evaluate a recent report which showed that city dwellers in India have 400 percent more heart disease than Americans? And almost half of these Indians were life-long vegetarians.[10] It has been found that vegetarians have just as much hardening of the arteries.[11] Clearly, meat is not the issue. There are other dietary factors involved. What the newest research suggests is that those who consume greater amounts of fiber, fruit, and nuts[12] have the least heart disease and greatest longevity. Typically, but not always, vegetarians consume more of these beneficial foods. Meat-eaters would be well-advised to do the same.

VEGETARIAN SHORTCOMINGS

Vitamin B_{12}

The best argument offering proof that humans were designed to consume animal products involves our need for vitamin B_{12}. It is essential for blood and nerve development. A deficiency can lead not only to anemia but also to neuropsychiatric disorders and even to permanent neurological damage. Usable vitamin B_{12} is found only in animal foods, particularly meat, eggs, and dairy. It should be pointed out that B_{12} needs to be combined with calcium in order to achieve proper utilization.[13] Vegans are usually advised to supplement with a B_{12}-containing yeast or with other foods supplemented with it because obtaining this vitamin from plant foods cannot be relied upon.

Long-term vegans, not careful to supplement, are at great risk of having a B_{12} deficiency; it can take years for symptoms to appear after stores of this nutrient have been exhausted. It is especially important for vegan lactating mothers to consume B_{12} supplements in order to avoid the grave effects a deficiency can have on the young child.[14,15] However, some folks are not even aware they have a deficiency if their diet is very high in folic acid. This part of the vitamin-B complex can mask anemic symptoms while permitting the underlying deficiency to wreak havoc.

Vitamin B_{12} helps to fight the effects of homocysteine. Without sufficient amounts of B_{12}, therefore, heart disease, stroke, and Alzheimer's disease due to high homocysteine levels may be more likely in a vegetarian diet.[16] In addition, a low output of hydrochloric acid (HCl) can interfere with absorption. A poorly functioning thyroid also can inhibit proper absorption of this important nutrient.[17] Unfortunately, many vegans rely on large amounts of soy for their protein, and soy has been shown to inhibit thyroid function. Not only that, even though fermented soy is the safest of soy products, many vegans rely on it, thinking that it is a non-animal source of vitamin B_{12}. However, the type of B_{12} in tempeh and miso (and sea vegetables as well) is the inactive form. These analogues of B_{12} compete in the body against any existing stores of the active form, thereby making a B_{12} deficiency worse. Animal sources seem to make the most sense. Perhaps this is why the Japanese rely so heavily on eggs to provide them with an excellent source of this vitamin. Dr. Stephen Byrnes, author, naturopath, and nutritionist claims to have saved two gentlemen from death due to anemia by getting them to eat a diet rich in dairy products. The two men had unfortunately felt that their vitamin B_{12} needs were being met by tempeh and spirulina.[18]

Iodine

If dairy products, seafood, or sea vegetables are not part of the diet, or if iodized salt is strictly limited, a deficiency of iodine can occur. Such deficiency can impact the thyroid which depends upon adequate supplies of this mineral. With diminished intakes of iodine, the thyroid-stimulating hormone (TSH) increases. This leads to the chance of developing hypothyroid conditions (weight gain, lack of energy, etc.)—or goiter. It has been found that a vegan diet may not supply enough iodine in the diet;

TSH levels were significantly higher in the vegan subjects—even in some of those who took kelp supplements—compared to those men consuming an omnivorous diet.[19] The research suggests, then, that vegans might become even more susceptible to the thyroid-damaging effects of soy, as well as to the goitrogens found in otherwise healthy foods they are likely to consume: broccoli, almonds, radishes, cabbage, rutabagas, mustard greens, kale, millet, cauliflower, turnips, pine nuts and peanuts. Infants, consuming large amounts of soy without the benefits of fish and dairy, also appear likely to suffer one of the consequences of hypothyroidism: reduced growth rates.[20]

Omega-3 Fatty Acids

When looking at the diets of the past that supported good health, it was found that the foods consumed had high levels of the omega-3 fatty acids in relation to the amounts of the other essential fatty acids, the omega-6s. Today, however, the general population is consuming far too many of the omega-6s from vegetable oils, largely because of the propaganda spread by the edible oil companies that consumption of these polyunsaturates will lead to better health. This problem is compounded by the fact that today's livestock is usually fed grains instead of grasses, causing the meat to lose much of its omega-3 content. These factors combine to upset a healthy balance between the two classes of fats. Even though nuts and seeds are among our best foods, the high levels of omega-6s can contribute to an imbalance if not enough omega-3s are consumed. Research continues to show how bringing the balance in line with the addition of omega-3 fatty acids may help with such conditions as hypertension, diabetes, and arthritis—the very conditions that plague modern society. The anti-inflammatory action of these fatty acids seems to be a key to their success in creating good health, especially for the heart.

Omega-3s (EPA and DHA) are found in coldwater fish and fish oils. Healthy cultures today still thrive when fish becomes an integral part of the diet—like the Japanese. Much of today's fish, unfortunately, if not contaminated by heavy metals and other pollutants, particularly in the larger predatory species, is farm-raised. The fatty-acid composition of these fish is negatively impacted as a result of the grains that are fed to them. And like the cattle feed-lots of today, these farm-raised fish are given antibiotics and growth-stimulating hormones. These fish are exposed to toxic chemicals, some of which are used to treat parasites that develop as a result of crowded living conditions. The fish are even treated with coloring chemicals to change the unhealthy gray color they develop into a red that we associate with wild fish.

Many people today have decided to consume only wild salmon or sardines which are not greatly impacted by mercury contamination. For their omega-3 intake other individuals are choosing to use only fish oil capsules or cod liver oil. Where does this leave the vegetarian who chooses to avoid even these healthy products? Flax, most likely.

Although flax seeds and their oil do not technically contain the valuable fish oils EPA and DHA, the fatty acid in flax (ALA) can be converted to them in the body, but only to a limited extent. It is estimated that only about 15–20 percent of the ALA is changed into the fish-type omega-3s. It may be for this reason that some studies using ALA have not been as successful in treating conditions that fish oils more readily handle. A diet high in omega-6 polyunsaturated oils and in *trans* fatty acids—as well as compromised health and older age—also limits the body's ability to effectively utilize the ALA in flax (and in walnuts). Perhaps those who are suited to the vegetarian lifestyle are those who have a greater ability to convert ALA.

This is not meant to knock flax. It is a tremendously valuable food, although the oil loses its protective abilities when heated. The ALA in flax and the fiber in the seed seem to have protective abilities beyond the fish oil considerations. Flax consumption has been associated with improved immune function, tumor inhibition, less heart disease and stroke, and it has been shown to improve male sexual function by virtue of its positive effect on testosterone. Vegetarians, however, may need to consume very high quantities of flax in order to receive the additional benefits from smaller amounts of wild, deep-water fish or fish oils. Both flax and fish promote health.

Vitamin A

Both vitamin A and beta carotene promote health as well. Vitamin A from butterfat, organ meat, shellfish, and egg yolks—and beta carotene from certain colorful fruits and vegetables appear to have beneficial effects independent of one another—even though beta carotene can be converted to vitamin A (retinol). These substances act as antioxidants; they protect the heart, fight cancer, fight infection, and promote healthy skin, eyes, bones, and intestinal-tract functioning.

Strict vegetarians who consume no preformed vitamin A from animal foods, even though they benefit from the beta carotene in their diet, run the risk of vitamin A deficiency if their bodies do not convert enough beta carotene into vitamin A. Diet researcher Dr. Price found that healthy, isolated peoples throughout the world ate ten times the amount of vitamin A from animal foods than today's typical American.[21] Many children and diabetics, as well as those with poor thyroid function, cannot make the proper conversion from beta carotene to vitamin A.[22] Furthermore, a low-fat diet adds to the problem since carotenes cannot be converted into vitamin A without the presence of fats in the diet.[23] Again, both plant and animal foods are supportive of good health.

Zinc

Zinc deficiencies are quite extensive in vegetarian populations—and in much of the general public as well. Zinc oversees many bodily processes and is particularly valuable for maintaining not only healthy prostate function, but also a healthy immune system. It helps regulate blood-sugar levels and is essential for proper mental functioning. Zinc deficiency during pregnancy can cause birth defects.[24]

It exists in substantial amounts in seafood, meat, and poultry, so if vegetarians are not supplementing with this vital nutrient, or not gobbling handfuls of pumpkin seeds, they are at a high risk of suffering from numerous problems. Although zinc can be found in grains and legumes, the phytic acid present in these foods can bind to and limit the amount of zinc absorbed by the body.

Vitamin D

This vitamin, which acts more like a hormone in the body, promotes growth, strong bones, and healthy teeth. Its ability to fight cancer is recently gaining more attention from researchers. Its sources are like those of vitamin A—animal foods. For those not eating these foods, supplements are available. But synthetic vitamin D_2 has been linked to hyperactivity and coronary heart disease, and synthetic D_3, that which is added to fortify milk, is poorly absorbed.[25] This leaves the vegetarian with the option of converting sunlight on the skin (in the presence of cholesterol) into vitamin D. Assuming that one does not slather the skin with sunscreens, adequate—not excessive—sunlight may be the most beneficial way to receive this nutrient. Unfortunately, a good number of Americans are either afraid of the sun or do not have the time to spend a portion of the day absorbing rays. People living in the northern latitudes have an even harder time getting enough sunlight to produce adequate amounts of vitamin D, a problem that is compounded by a vegetarian diet.[26]

Many Americans are deficient due to either limited sun exposure or lack of sunlight during winter months—vegetarians and nonvegetarians alike. Although it is quite possible to overdose on vitamin D, particularly if you are getting plenty of sunshine and simultaneously consume cod liver oil, it now appears that the need for this substance is much greater than what is currently recommended. Again, this greater amount makes sense in terms of the high levels of vitamin D that Dr. Price found were consumed by healthy cultures. Without the sunlight, without the eggs and butter, and without the seafood or cod liver oil, it is no wonder that long-term vegetarians have a difficult time keeping osteoporosis at bay.[27,28]

Protein

Animal foods provide complete protein—that is, protein containing all of the essential amino acids necessary for the body's proper maintenance, growth, and energy needs. If there is sufficient hydrochloric acid to digest this protein, it can also support the immune system and maintain proper blood-sugar levels. Vegetarians who are careful in their food choices can achieve proper protein levels by mixing and matching vegetable sources of protein which, when consumed alone, are not quite complete. However, many of them choose to do so with soy because it most closely resembles the amino-acid profile of animal products, with the exception of being deficient in essential methionine and low in lysine, compared to milk protein. Relying solely on soy for one's protein needs is not a good idea. Besides being deficient in the valuable A and D vitamins, soy, like other legumes, contains some tannin and plenty of trypsin inhibitors that interfere with the breakdown of protein into the valuable amino acids. Trypsin is an enzyme that accomplishes the breakdown task. There-fore, the amino acids from soy protein are not as available to the body when compared to those obtained from animal protein.[29] The same holds true with regard to the absorption of a number of key minerals such as iron, magnesium, and phosphorus.[30,31]

It has been said that "you are what you eat." Others have been more insightful and have claimed that "you are what you digest." Since protein from soy (and plant protein in general) is more difficult to digest than animal protein, the undigested protein can create health problems of its own by virtue of its causal relationship to allergies. The leading authority on soy trypsin inhibitors, Irwin Leiner, Ph.D., Professor Emeritus from the University of Minnesota, believes that particular soy proteins, lectins, interfere with growth because they inhibit the use of essential nutrients. He believes, as well, that the soy trypsin inhibitors retard growth and lead to a loss of protein. He suggested in a letter to the FDA that we not dis-miss the possibility that "soybean trypsin inhibitors do, in fact, pose a potential risk to humans when soy protein is incorporated into the diet."[32,33]

VEGETARIAN EXCESSES

Grain Carbohydrates

Nutritionist Robert Crayhon points out that a 1997 study appearing in the *American Journal of Clinical Nutrition* concluded that "there is now substantial evidence that low-fat, high-carbohydrate diets lead to changes in glucose, insulin, and lipoprotein metabolism that will increase the risk of ischemic heart disease."[34] Partly because of the popularity of the work of Dr. Atkins, Americans are becoming more aware that a diet too high in carbohydrates, especially the refined ones, can lead to numerous problems beyond heart disease. Fluctuating blood-sugar levels can lead to energy imbalances, food-cravings, and the overeating of even more carbohydrates. A vicious cycle is established in which weight gain is often inevitable. Yeast overgrowths and gluten intolerance are also associated with a diet high in grains; these conditions can lead to fatigue, bloating, infections, depression, diarrhea, malabsorption of vitamins, neurological problems and worse. An increased risk of breast and colorectal cancers is associated with diets high in bread and cereal products.[35] The savvy vegetarian will try to limit grain carbohydrate and focus on the veggies for a source of carbs and for fiber.

Phytates

Most well-read vegetarians are aware that, if consuming cereal grains, whole-grain products should be eaten rather than the simple, refined carbohydrates because of their ability to prevent blood-sugar spikes. But a heavy reliance on whole grains can have its own set of problems. Some whole grains have been puffed to make rice cakes. Not only does this process make the whole grain even more damaging to insulin balance than pure sugar,[36] it creates toxic elements that have caused rapid death in test animals.[37] Even the typical boxed, extruded, whole-grain cereals have been processed at such high temperatures that, not only are many nutrients destroyed, but the adverse effects on blood sugar are more damaging than pure sugar.[38] The U.S. Food and Drug Administration, however, recently authorized the cereal companies to promote the cancer and heart-disease-fighting health benefits of cereals like Cheerios and Wheaties.

Like most grains, these whole-grain cereals contain phytic acid (phytates). Phytic acid binds to a number of minerals like calcium, magnesium, zinc, and iron and make them less available to the body. Since strict vegetarians often do not obtain enough calcium (from dairy products), and inject more grain and legume phytates, they may be at greater risk for decreased bone mineral density.[39] This problem is exacerbated by the fact that most grains are acid-forming foods which, like very high-protein/low-carbohydrate diets,[40] attempt to pull additional calcium from the bones.

Phytic acid is useful in small amounts by virtue of its ability to bind to potentially dangerous heavy metals. Too much iron, for example, can have devastating effects—heart disease and cancer—but many vegetarians unfortunately find themselves iron-deficient. Refined carbohydrates with the phytates removed and with extra iron purposely added to make up for the refining process may, on the other hand, create an iron overload for those consuming too many of these sugary-type carbs. In short, mineral deficiencies are likely in a vegetarian diet if too many whole grains (and legumes) are consumed. One or two servings of grains per day are more conducive to good health than the six to eleven per day recommended by the USDA food pyramid.

A major source of carbohydrates in the Japanese diet, of course, is rice—served at most meals. Much of the rice consumed is white. At first, it seems odd that the Japanese, who are generally regarded as having healthy diets, would resort to using this refined grain since it is so inferior to brown rice. The following might explain this puzzling situation: Similar to how Westerners began to use refined sugar and flour because of their association with purity and the upper class, Asians began very long ago to mimic their nobility who consumed white rice that was painstakingly polished by hand. Already revered as a food that represents life and fertility (accounting for the ritual of throwing it at weddings), white rice also became a symbol for wealth and, therefore, very desirable.

Any food, no matter how nutritious, however, can present problems if it is eaten in excess. As a staple food in Japan, brown rice is no different. The phytic acid present in this whole grain has the potential to deplete important minerals. Ironically, then, the switch to polished rice, though depriving the population of important B and E vitamins, may prevent the loss of certain minerals if brown rice were heavily consumed instead. Apparently, an otherwise diverse Japanese diet makes up for the nutrients missing in the polished rice, although one wonders about the problems created by consuming the talc which is often added to white rice. Westerners, of course, are advised to consume brown rice, but only in moderation as part of a varied diet. Asians appear to be genetically better able to consume greater amounts of grains. Enzyme expert and pioneer, Edward Howell, claims that Asians have a substantially heavier pancreas and larger salivary glands that secrete an enzyme (amylase) responsible for the digestion of carbohydrates. This would make Asians better suited to a vegetarian diet, although strict vegetarianism appears to be rare in Japan.

Grains can be an important component of a healthful diet. Not only has consumption of whole grains been associated with improved insulin response and with lower rates of certain cancers, grain-eating has been linked with a 15–25 percent reduction in ischemic heart disease. The best results were in those (postmenopausal women) who consumed just one or two servings a day.[41] It's the matter of overconsumption that should be on the mind of vegetarians and nonvegetarians alike. Traditional cultures often countered the problem with grain and legume phytates by soaking, sprouting, or fermenting them before consumption. Such handling of these foods also reduces the amount of enzyme inhibitors they contain that interfere with digestion and nutrient absorption. Soaking brown rice several hours before cooking, for example, makes this grain even more nutritious.

Lectins

The study of lectins and their effect on human health is a relatively new science. What are lectins? They are carbohydrate-binding proteins found in most plant foods.

Some of them are toxic and inflammatory and are notably found in foods consumed in large amounts by vegetarians: soy and wheat. In fact, wheat may be the most overconsumed food in the country. These lectins are suspected of binding to the gut wall and changing gut permeability, a condition commonly known as "leaky gut syndrome." Incidentally, cholesterol maintains the health of the intestinal wall.[42] With greater gut permeability, lectins and other substances that are best kept out of the bloodstream can eventually circulate to various organs and may create autoimmune responses. Rheumatoid arthritis, insulin-dependent diabetes, kidney disease, peptic ulcers, lupus, and celiac disease are all thought to have dietary lectins as a possible cause. For celiac disease, gluten (as in wheat) avoidance is a standard treatment.

Lectins also appear to strip away the mucus lining that forms a barrier that protects the upper respiratory tract. This loss of mucus makes a person more susceptible to a number of infectious agents. Allergist David L. Freed suggests that the "stone-age/paleolithic diet"—a diet free of most of these toxic grain and starchy toxic lectins—may protect against some common viral infections. Why, then, are we all not sick? Almost all of us are consuming dietary lectins. Could it be the quantity we consume? The hunter–gather populations obtained from 56–65 percent of their calories from animal sources and thrived.[43,44] Dr. Freed suggests that perhaps our guts offer a natural protection to lectins. A fine screen of sialic acid molecules seems to prevent the lectins from creating harm, but these molecules can be stripped away by certain viruses, making us vulnerable.[45] Others have suggested that the use of aspirin and other anti-inflammatory medications may also weaken our resistance to lectins.

OTHER PROBLEMS

Vegetarians have been found to be deficient not only in the important amino acid taurine and the amino-like nutrient carnitine, but also in the cancer-fighting mineral selenium. Additionally, a diet high in grains interferes with the activity of the B vitamin biotin. Both biotin and carnitine are essential for healthy fat metabolism.[46] Whether it is these deficiencies—or the numerous ones previously mentioned—there is something about a vegetarian diet that appears to be linked to a troubling birth defect—hypospadia. It has been reported that vegetarian mothers are five times more likely to give birth to sons with a penis defect.[47]

Researchers are puzzled. The cause may not be a nutrient deficiency but perhaps something additional in the diet that is affecting the endocrine system. Could it be that vegetarian mothers who are not careful to eat organically are consuming too many hormone-disrupting pesticides? Or is it all the unfermented soy? A heavy consumption of soy phytoestrogens by the pregnant mother is suspected by some of interfering with the proper sexual development of the young boy. Much still needs to be learned.

ENVIRONMENTAL CONCERNS

Vegetarians concerned about the economic, social, and environmental aspects of consuming meat warn us that it typically takes several pounds of grains to yield just one pound of meat—not at all an efficient use of resources. These grains, we are told, could otherwise be used to feed the world's starving population. We are also warned that acres upon acres of rain forest are cut down yearly to support livestock. The transportation of meat over long distances uses up a disproportionately high amount of fossil fuels. Giant feed lots use huge amounts of water and create tons of waste that pollute our waterways. All seemingly true.

On the other hand, a reliance on the giant, monocultured crops of today's agribusiness (vast acres of a single plant) creates fields of nutrient-depleted soils which are then "perked-up" with artificial fertilizers made from petrochemicals. Some of these fields receive as many as ten applications of pesticides and fungicides manufactured from even more fuel sources. Much of this grain is used to feed livestock and carries these poisons into the meat and milk of the animal. The pesticide contamination of drinking water from field run-off or from water-table exposure creates a health risk to many, not to mention the exposure farm workers receive from applying these toxins. Fish caught in most of the nation's pesticide-polluted bays are not suitable for consumption.

The public is becoming more aware of these serious problems. The increased frequency with which organic produce and other products are appearing in markets is encouraging. Even though organic foods represent only 1 percent of total food sales, giant agribusiness interests, however, appear to be showing concern about this growing trend. Attempting to instill fear in the public over relying on organic food, Dennis T. Avery has recently written an article about the purported "dangers" of organic produce. His work appeared not only in *The Wall Street Journal*, but was also picked up by the Associated Press and distributed widely.

Among his claims is that organic food is much more likely to be contaminated with deadly *E. coli* as a result of the manure often used in organic farming: "Organic foods have clearly become the deadliest food choice."[48] The only thing that is clear is that Mr. Avery has no evidence whatsoever to back up his claims. His statistics were invented.[49] It appears that Mr. Avery also spreads plenty of manure.

By the way, Dennis Avery's employer, the Hudson Institute, is "a free-market, proglobalization think tank" that has reportedly received funding from the likes of Monsanto, Du Pont, DowElanco, Sandoz, and Ciba-Geigy, as well as agribusiness giants ConAgra, Cargill, and Procter & Gamble. The Hudson Institute previously published a book written by Mr. Avery titled: *Saving the Planet with Pesticides and Plastic*. Enough said?

No, it must also be pointed out that not only is organic food free of many potentially harmful chemicals, but a review of the literature collected during the last 50 years on this topic has found organically grown food to be nutritionally superior to that which is conventionally grown.[50] Animal studies have even shown "better growth and reproduction in animals fed organically grown feed compared with those fed conventionally grown feed."[51]

A BETTER WAY

Most current farming practices, whether it's by the meat industry or by the grain/legume conglomerates, are abysmal. Both are detrimental to the environment. We need not be forced to choose between the two. There is another way. We need to return to the most productive and environmentally friendly way of feeding the population: the mixed farm. Organic farmer and dairyman Mark Purdey tells us that a well-managed farm that grows a number of different crops and raises a variety of livestock keeps the land and soil healthy without the use of synthetic toxins and fertilizers. The recycling of materials (vegetable waste, cow poop, etc.) and proper crop rotation keep the soil vital. The animals can eat plant material grown on the farm. Chickens can peck and scavenge, and cattle can be free to roam and eat the clover and other sources of high-protein forage from unfertile grassland. Such management of natural resources can provide four harvests per season compared to only one or two from the typical monocropped acres.[52]

Buying from a variety of local farms would reduce fuel consumption involved with cross-country transportation. There would be less use of grain to feed the cows. Besides, cows are healthier on a grass diet, and the milk and meat they produce are healthier for us, too. By the way, the argument that feeding grains to animals takes that food out of the mouths of the unfortunate ones in third-world countries does not hold up. There is already enough food to feed everyone in the world. The problem is with distribution, wars, and politics. In India, for example, there is a glut of food in the government's possession. Some of it is exported, and some of it is rotting in storehouses while half of the country's children under four are malnourished, and 60 percent of the country's women are anemic.[53]

Most of the acreage in this country is not suitable for agriculture. There are countless acres of rocky or hilly, nutrient-poor land. There are square miles of unfertile grassland suited for nothing better than the raising of livestock. Buffalo meat from such land is extremely nutritious, as the American Indians of long ago knew so well. Acres of forests do not need to be cut down. Since small farms may not be able to meet all the meat needs of an entire nation, utilizing this unfarmable land for livestock grazing makes the best use of this resource. We simply don't need or want those giant feed lots. Enig and Fallon point out: "It is not animal cultivation that leads to hunger and famine but unwise agricultural practices and monopolistic distribution systems."[54]

Farmer (and scientist) Mark Purdey also decries today's food industry. It is controlled by too few, and it is too wasteful. There is little thought given to the environment and little care given to the animals. Mr. Purdey longs for a comeback of the type of small, mixed farms he first saw many years ago in England:

> All of the farms and their staff seemed vibrant with the ethereal relationship flowing between the soil, the crops, the livestock and the landscape. My life metamorphosed effortlessly into higher dimensions, eternally flavoured by the mantra of the mixed farm. By day, bull finches and bees droned through orchards like an avant-garde orchestra; hens scuttled in random syncopation

beneath the boughs, scuffling up the dust in the nettlebeds and churning up the aromatic incense of the earth before the rain came. Evenings were fanned by the wings of horseshoe bats, cockchaffers and chiffchaffs. Dusks drifted into nights screech-scouted by barn owls presiding over rickyards, linhays and looseboxes all bursting with a lava flow of manure; the mainstay of global well-being.[55]

■■ **TIPS:** ■■

Consume two or three servings a day of gluten-free whole grains or sprouted wheat bread.

Be aware that puffed and processed "whole" grains are not rich in nutrients and may cause insulin spikes.

Avoid soy milk and tofu as main protein sources.

Vegetarians need to be certain to get enough zinc and vitamin D. Zinc can be acquired by eating pumpkin seeds; vitamin D by eating organ meats, seafood, and dairy products. Adequate sunlight will provide the necessary vitamin D, and most people can benefit from cod liver oil, which contains valuable vitamin A as well.

Supplement with a high-quality flax seed oil, or fresh, refrigerated, organic flax seeds. The seeds should be ground just before use for maximum benefit.

THE BEST DIET

IS THERE ONE?

No, there isn't a "best diet." We should all know this. We know that everyone possesses a unique "biochemical individuality." We can make broad generalizations about nutrients essential for optimal health, but to assume that all humans have the same basic nutritional requirements is a mistake. One nationally recognized author who has written several low-fat diet books (along with the help of his wife) was heard to say on his radio talk show that, like dog food, there is just one proper type of people food (meaning: a vegan diet).

How silly. He may even be wrong about the dog food. A one-size-fits-all approach doesn't work. Yet we continue to flock to the latest new or recycled diet, whatever the current trend is, whether it's a Mediterranean diet, a Zone diet, an Ornish diet, or an Atkins diet. We want the quick fix. We want results. We want someone to give us the answers. We will abandon the common-sense notion that we have our own individual dietary needs in favor of participating in the latest diet fad. We want to identify with something outside ourselves—with a group, whether it's a political party or a religion—or Weight Watchers. We want to belong to something that we hope will further define us—a quick fix to discover who we are.

Some of us have begun to compromise. Recognizing that to some extent we are indeed different from one another, but still wanting a label that will define our specific eating needs, we have opted for a number of diet plans that match our body "type." This could be a blood type, a metabolic type, an ethnic/ancestral type, or even an Ayurvedic body type (constitution). This is still the quick-fix approach, but at least we are headed in the right direction.

CREATING A MATCH

The recent popularity of matching foods to our blood type (ABO) seems well-deserved, at first glance. If we are type A then a vegetarian diet may be suitable for us, we are told. If we are type O, the oldest blood type, then our bodies are better designed to eat meat, and so on. Unfortunately, blood typing is just too broad—kind of like astrology—not specific enough.

Nutritional expert and author Alan Gaby, M.D., claims that ABO typing is just one way to identify blood. According to Dr. Gaby there are more than thirty unique markers on the surface of red blood cells, plus many more on white blood cells. "It is likely that a diet based on the ABO system would be completely different than one based on another set of markers."[1] If one wishes to base diet on blood typing, it might be necessary to choose from among 40 or 50 diets, each matching a specific blood marker. Science isn't there yet.

Ancient Ayurvedic medicine from India offers another way to help us chose the right diet. Simply establish what body type (dosha) you are from your basic physical and temperamental traits, and then choose from a list of foods that are most conducive to health for your dosha. If you are considered to be a "vata," then eating beef is fine. If you are a "pitta" or "kapha," then it is a no-no. What would you do if you are a kapha as well as a "meat-eating" blood type O?

There are centuries of science behind Ayurvedic medicine. It is not to be scoffed at. Unfortunately, a system that has worked well for over 4000 years in India—with its rather homogeneous population—is unlikely to work as well with the ethnic and physical diversity (melting pot) we have in today's America.

Another system of matching diet to body type is that which was developed in the 1970s by Dr. William Kelly. He felt that blood type was not a significant factor. He recognized that we are indeed all different, but for him the key differences were in the nervous system categories (sympathetic or parasympathetic). Dr. Kelly felt it essential to rebalance the nervous system through diet. To that end he developed diets for ten metabolic "types," taking into consideration, almost in an Ayurvedic fashion, one's personality, physiology, and neurological makeup. Again, if everyone has a different metabolic and nervous system profile, it is difficult to see how we all can neatly fit into specific groups—ten in this case. It's a nice, round number.

TWO BASIC GROUPS?

Some nutritionists today are attempting to simplify matters by putting us into two basic groups: "fast burners and slow burners." This sounds good. If you burn your food rapidly, then fat and protein from meat are for you (to balance the speed of the energy conversion). If you are a slow metabolizer, on the other hand, then keep fat intake to a minimum and avoid the simple carbohydrates because of your inherent problem with blood sugar and insulin levels. Is there such a thing as a "medium-burner"? If so, can you eat whatever you want?

Does the speed at which you metabolize food primarily depend on, as Kelly suggests, your nervous system, or does it rely on other factors? There is plenty of evidence to suggest that the type of fat your body possesses (brown fat or white fat) influences metabolism. If your body contains a large amount of brown fat, the cells of which have a greater concentration of energy-producing mitochondria, then many of your food calories will be converted to heat instead of to fat. If you don't have much brown fat, which is concentrated in the neck and back, weight gain is likely to be your reward. How much brown fat do you have?

TOO MANY CHOICES

So what are we to do? There may be grains of truth in all of these diet systems. Do we try them all out, one at a time? Or mix several together? Perhaps we find our blood type, our metabolic type, our dosha—see what foods are permitted for each—and if we're lucky we might find something worthwhile to eat. Instead, maybe we should consider our ancestral background and eat like they did. Do you know what your ancestors ate? Do you even truly know your ancestral heritage? Many in this country do not.

The head spins with so much to consider—but only because we have bought into the quick-fix, easy-answer concept to our nutritional dilemma. What we have lost sight of is how our biochemical individuality expresses itself and how the food we eat affects us. We have simply lost touch with ourselves.

We have blindly accepted what the advertisers and public health officials have told us—and what the diet guru of the day tells us. We have been told not to worry, just eat like the food pyramid shows. You know how it's laid out—low fat (low even in the healthy fats), with the heaviest emphasis on carbohydrates without distinguishing between the fiber-rich whole grains and the nutrient-poor, blood-sugar-raising, white flour products.

Walter Willett, chair of the Department of Nutrition at the Harvard School of Public Health, explains that the food pyramid is built on "shaky scientific grounds."[2] It was of course developed by the U.S. Department of Agriculture whose allegiance is not to public health but to the well-being of the farming community.

Professor Willett has taken note of the fact that one investigation of the large, ongoing Nurses Health Study found that those who followed the government food pyramid were no healthier than those who didn't. As a consequence, rates of cancer and heart disease remain high. Hypothyroidism, diabetes, and obesity are rampant. And osteoporosis continues to cripple. (See pp. 132–133 for a superior—and flexible—replacement for the USDA Food Pyramid.)

LOOKING INWARD

We are less healthy today because we no longer look inward to find the "best diet." We continue to look outside for the answers. We view our bodies as boxes or tubes: Put in the "right" food and get the "right" result. The truth is, we are more than boxes. The mind–body connection must not be overlooked. With medications, the placebo effect shows that our minds affect how we react to what enters our bodies. It appears to be no different with food. According to Rene Dubos, one of the foremost scientists and thinkers of the twentieth century, as well as one of the earliest promoters of biochemical individuality: "It takes more than a knowledge of foodstuffs to create a science of human nutrition."[3]

Author and researcher Larry Dossey agrees: "It's often the eater, not what's eaten, that matters most. . . . a physically based, formulaic approach that leaves no room for our emotional and spiritual life has no hope in succeeding." This conclusion is illustrated by Dr. Dossey in the November 1998 issue of *Alternative Therapies in Health and Medicine* with two fascinating examples. He writes:

> In a study of a large group of beggars in India, all of them were found to pursue a diet that had long been deficient in calories; iron; calcium; phosphorus; vitamins A, B, C, and D; and animal protein. To their astonishment, the researchers discovered that only 4% of the beggars showed obvious signs of nutritional deficiency, and radiographic studies showed most of them having a normally calcified skeleton. Among the female beggars, the diet had no markedly deleterious effect on either pregnancy or lactation, and the growth rate of children in the group was only slightly lower than normal.[4]

Can the decent health of these individuals be explained by the human body adapting to poor nutritional intake? Or could there be another explanation—a spiritual/emotional connection? Could food have the ability to be either a positive or a negative force in our lives, depending on the emotional context in which it is consumed? Dossey's second example is even more illuminating.

He describes an experiment in which rabbits were fed a diet high in fat and cholesterol. After the animals were killed and examined, it was found as predicted, since rabbits cannot handle such a diet, that there were obstructions and ulcerations in the arteries such as those that would lead to heart attacks in humans. However, one specific group of rabbits demonstrated atherosclerotic changes that were 60 percent less than those of the overall group. The investigators were astonished.

It was eventually discovered that the rabbits less affected were cared for by one of the investigators who, during the course of the experiment, regularly took the rabbits from their cages and petted, stroked, and talked to them. To discover whether this was just a coincidence, another study began in which two groups of rabbits were fed the same high-fat diet, but one group was removed from the cages several times a day to be given petting and attention, each time by the same person. The results: again 60 percent lower incidence of atherosclerosis in the handled group.

The experiment was then repeated. The results were the same in all three experiments. According to Dossey, "Touching, petting, handling, and gentle talking emerged as a crucial determinant in the disease process that kills more Americans than any other."

FOOD AND EMOTIONS

Much publicity has surrounded the work of Dr. Dean Ornish in which a diet that minimizes fat intake can actually reverse the initial stages of heart disease. What is not so commonly known, however, according to nutritionist Robert Crayhon, is that the low-fat aspect of his treatment was just one of five ways to treat heart disease. Besides diet, there were four other lifestyle changes involved: stopping smoking, moderate aerobic exercise, stress management, and group support.[5] In light of what Dossey and others suspect, the low-fat diet may have very little to do with reversing heart disease. Positive emotions combined with a reverence and appreciation for our food may be the key factor that unleashes food's power to nurture.

Emotions simply cannot be overlooked. In America, there is often too much dietary conflict. Frequent guests at our breakfast and dinner tables include confusion, guilt, worry, and fear about the food we are eating. These traits can certainly have a negative impact on our digestion and, quite likely, the way our bodies regard the nutrients. Many of the people in France, apparently, do not have this problem. The rarity of heart disease there, despite high-fat diets, has been attributed either to copious amounts of red wine or to a high consumption of fresh fruits and vegetables—or to a disdain for fast foods. Psychology professor Dr. Paul Rozin notes, however: "The French have no ambivalence about food: it's almost purely a source of pleasure."[6]

Perhaps it is this emotional context that ultimately makes food a sustainer of life instead of a killer. Sadly, if Americans are not obsessing or worrying about their food, then too many of them are eating on the run, having little social context with their meals apart from the nightly news, or they eat to fill an emotional emptiness or to soothe chronic distress. In short, we are largely unconscious about our food. It is this point that is addressed beautifully by a number of writers including Marc David in his book *Nourishing Wisdom*. He notes that: "Eating is a vastly unexplored area in psychology. . . . Unlike animals who *feed*, humans beings *eat*. That is, food for us is largely cultural and psychological rather than instinctual."[7]

It is our attitude and awareness about the food we eat that can play an important role in health. We need to become more conscious not only of what we eat, but also why we eat. Many of us are unconscious about what is happening within. Perhaps introspection is genetically based—a skill or trait not all possess or can possess. Let us hope not.

AWARENESS AND CHANGE

An example of how we have come to be out of touch with our bodies involves a simple thing like water. Some studies suggest that a huge percentage of the population is chronically dehydrated. We may not be fully aware of the strong diuretic effects of coffee, tea, and alcohol. We experience thirst and then drink more of the same stuff. We fail to ask, "How much water have I actually had today?" And as we continue to become further dehydrated, our bodies often mistake this sensation for hunger. So we eat, although we don't need the food. Eventually weight gain ensues and we continue to have a water deficit. We've lost touch. We are out of tune. And our health suffers because we don't pay attention.

We know that the body changes constantly. As we age we may require greater amounts of nutrients like carnitine or CoQ10—substances our bodies begin to produce in decreasing amounts. Some of us may need more hydrochloric acid to digest food properly as we age. We must adapt over time to our bodies' changes. However, conscious eating means keeping up with the changes we experience moment by moment. We are not the same person we were the day before. We may look the same, but the continual chemical ebb and flow linked to our neurological apparatus makes us new beings not just each day, but rather each second of the day. (In one second alone, millions of red blood cells are born and die.)

To address those changes and become more aware of our eating, Mr. David suggests asking this before putting anything into your mouth:

Am I hungry?
Will food satisfy my hunger?
What would truly nourish me in this moment?
Do I choose to eat?

EAT LIKE A MAN (A CAVEMAN)

Some fortunate people are able to perceive the correct signals from the body which, when listened to, will tell us what to eat—as well as how much. Others need a little help to get started on the path to conscious eating in order to attain better health. We know the importance of avoiding the toxins in foods. We know to eat pesticide-free food whenever possible and to avoid damaged fats and oils. We also are aware that our diets should limit sugar and white flour products, relying instead on whole, natural, unrefined foods. But which ones?

A look at how humans have eaten for over two million years offers a good starting point. From a genetic standpoint, we are essentially the same as our paleolithic ancestors who evolved eating what has been called a "caveman" or "hunter–gatherer" diet. Our bodies have developed to efficiently process the nutrients from foods eaten during these countless years. It is therefore suggested that our nutritional needs depend more on what was eaten then rather than what we typically consume today. What were those foods? Wild game of every type (making up over 50% of the calories), nuts and seeds, sometimes eggs, wild plants, and fruits in the warmer climates, and insects and worms.

This is a very short list, but it is how the human developed into a very robust creature—until about 10,000–15,000 years ago—when the "paleolithic" diet came largely to an end. According to Robert Crayhon, "This switch away from meat saw humans lose six inches in height, suffer a dramatic increase in tooth decay and bone malformations, suffer increased infant mortality, and acquire many diseases not known in hunter–gatherer groups such as adult onset diabetes and coronary heart disease."[8] This switch was to a new agricultural diet in which dairy products, grains, legumes, and beans were consumed.

It has been argued that our paleolithic ancestors simply died too early to have the chance to develop "modern" diseases and ailments. "This claim is simply false," say a number of experts, including author S. Boyd Eaton, who have studied the paleolithic diet and longevity.[9] Though our primitive ancestors did die frequently from accidents and infections, if they were able to escape these hazards, according to nutritionist Elson Haas, "their longevity was similar to ours, but with much less chronic degenerative disease."[10]

SIMPLIFY

It is suggested that 10,000 years is not long enough for most humans to adapt to this new diet. Most people in the world still are unable to digest cow's milk. Countless others have food sensitivities or allergies to grains, particularly to gluten-containing wheat, oats, rye, and barley. Yet these products permeate the modern diet and may be causing problems for many people. Nutrition and science consultant, Leigh Broadhurst, Ph.D., is quite adamant: "Virtually all chronic disease results from abandoning the Paleolithic diet."[11]

A number of cultures, however, have adapted to grain and dairy, and when not used in excess, these foods can offer considerable nutritional benefit. Therefore, by starting with a paleolithic or even a traditional ancestral diet, one can begin to add some of the "newer" foods, always remaining conscious of how the body accepts them.

If it has taken over 10,000 years just for some of us to be able to deal with grains, beans, and milk, think about how many new "foods" have been introduced to us during recent decades. And consider the countless food additives designed to improve shelf-life, color, texture, or flavor. Will humans ever be able to adapt without ill-effect to these substances (like MSG or sodium nitrite), whose safety has already been proven to be questionable at best? Or to the hydrogenated oil and hydrolyzed vegetable protein found in so many of today's foods?

Dr. Dossey tells us that American consumers in the 1920s had only a few hundred food products to choose from. By 1965 about 800 new products were being introduced each year, and in 1995 alone there were 16,863 new products on the market shelves!

Thoreau was right. We need to simplify in order to get back in tune with our bodies' needs. We can shop for food as if we were back in the 1920s or earlier—before heart disease began to take its grim toll. We can eat without the fear of natural fats found in traditional diets. Or we can start with a paleolithic-like diet. Emphasize organic fruits and vegetables, raw nuts and seeds (soaked or sprouted), and high-quality, hormone-free meat. Feel free to skip the insects and worms.

THE NONPYRAMID
FOOD GUIDE

The "Eating for Health" diagram on the next page was developed by Edward Bauman, Ph.D, director of the Institute for Educational Therapy (now Bauman College), a state-licensed vocational school that provides professional certification for nutrition consultants and natural chefs. It is based in Cotati, California.

Of special note is the central (bull's eye) importance of obtaining the essential fatty acids from nuts and seeds such as flax, walnuts, and almonds (best raw, soaked, or sprouted), as well as from the health-promoting olive and coconut oils—organic butter included.

Also noteworthy is the emphasis placed on obtaining adequate protein. Part of the beauty of this schematic is its flexibility. Those who have found that long-lasting health can be achieved on a vegan diet can obtain their protein from vegetable sources. The semi-vegetarians can be certain to add free-range eggs and organic dairy products. Those who fare well on other animal foods can meet their additional protein needs with grass-fed beef and buffalo, lamb, free-range chickens, and salmon (wild, not farm-raised).

Avoiding tap water with its chlorine and fluoride is a must. And it's time to dust off that juicer which you haven't used in years in order to benefit from the many vitamins and enzymes found in unpasteurized juices.

Eating 4 Health

Organic, **Seasonal**, Nutrient-rich, and Individualized

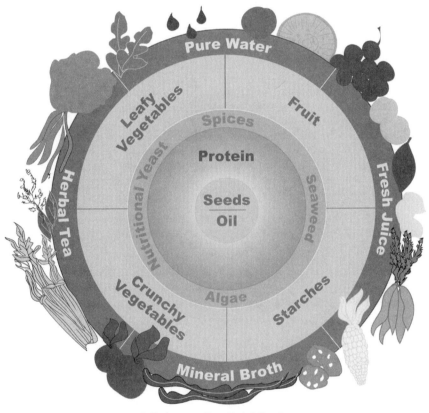

A Rejuvenating Food System
© Edward Bauman, Ph.D.

	Seeds/Oils	Protein	Leafy Vegetables	Crunchy Vegetables	Starches	Seasonal Fruit
Daily servings	2-3	2-4	1-3	1-3	2-4	2-4
Servings size	1 Tbs. oil 2 Tbs. seeds	3 oz. animal 6 oz. legume	1 cup	1/2 cup	1/2 c. root vegetable grains, bread	1/2 cup or 1 medium piece
Examples	Flax, sunflower, sesame, almonds	Poultry, fish, eggs, milk, beans	Salad mix, kale, spinach	Broccoli, string beans, cukes, onion, celery	Yams, winter squash, corn, millet, rice	Berries, apple, grape, citrus

The Institute for Educational Therapy offers the comprehensive, affordable and professional Nutrition Consultant and Natural Chef Training Programs in a classroom or distance learning format. For more information: www.iet.org / (800) 987-7530

Notes

Green Tea

1. "Dietary Reference Values"(1996), The Report of the Department of Health and Social Subjects, No. 41,Chapter 36 on fluoride, HMSO.
2. Marilyn Chase, article on R. Isaacson's "Rat Studies Link Brain Cell Damage with Aluminum and Fluoride in Water" (State University of New York, Binghamton) in *Wall Street Journal*, Oct. 28, 1992, p. B–6.
3. J. A. Varner, K. F. Jensen, W. Horvath, and R. L. Isaacson, "Chronic Administration of Aluminum-fluoride or Sodium-fluoride to Rats in Drinking Water: Alterations in Neuronal and Cerebrovascular Integrity," *Brain Research*, 1998, 784: 284–298.
4. G. N. Jenkins, "Fluoride Intake and Its Safety Among Heavy Tea Drinkers in a British Fluoridated City," *Proc Finn Dent Soc*, 1991, 87(4): 571–579.
5. A. Diouf, F. O. Sy, B. Niane, D. Ba, and M. Ciss, "Dietary Intake of Fluorine Through a Tea Prepared by the Traditional Method in Senegal," *Dakar Med*, 1994, 39(2): 227–30.
6. G. N. Opinya, N. Bwibo, J. Valderhaug, J. M. Birkeland, and P. Lokken, "Intake of Fluoride and Excretion in Mothers' Milk in a High Fluoride (9 ppm) Area in Kenya," *Eur J Clin Nutr*, 1991, 45(1): 37–41.
7. Andreas Schuld, www.bruha.com/fluoride/html/green_tea___f.html.
8. "Toxicological Profile for Fluorides, Hydrogen Fluoride and Fluorine" (1993), ATSDR/U.S. Public Health Service, p. 46, www.bruha.com/fluoride/html/green_tea___f.html.
9. B. Hileman, "Fluoridation of water. Questions about health risks and benefits remain after more than 40 years." *Chemical and Engineering News,* Aug. 1, 1988, pp. 26–42.
10. A. Singh et al., "Endemic fluorosis. Epidemiological, clinical and biochemical study of chronic fluoride intoxication in Pubjab." *Medicine,* 1963, 42: 229–246.
11. "Fluorides and Human Health" (1970), report by World Health Orginization, Geneva, Switzerland, pp. 32, 239–240.
12. http://www.fluoridealert.org/news/NYSCOF-osteoarthritis.htm.
13. P. M. Galetti and G. Joyet, "Effect of Fluorine On Thyroidal Iodine Metabolism in Hyperthyroidism," *J Clin Endocrinol*, 1958, 18: 1102–1110.
14. L. J. De Groot, P. Reed-Larsen, and G. Hennemann, eds., *The Thyroid and Its Diseases*, 6th ed., (New York: Churchill Livingstone, 1996). Chapter 18, revised 1 April 2001 by Furio Pacini.
15. S. Langer and J. Scheer, *Solved: The Riddle of Illness* (New Canaan, CT: Keats, 1984).
16. F. C. Whittelsey, "What's in Your Green Tea?" *In These Times*, August 21, 2000, http://www.inthesetimes.com/issue/24/19/whittelsey2419.html.
17. T. Sztarbala, R. Gos, J. Kedziora, J. Blaszczyk, E. Sibinska, and M. Goralczyk, "Changes in the Antioxidant System of the Vitreous in Rabbits after Administration of Sulfur Hexafluoride," *Klin Oczna*, 1998, 100(2): 69–71.
18. I. C. Arts, P. C. Hollman, and D. Kromhou, "Chocolate as a source of tea flavonoids," *Lancet*, 1999, 354: 488.
19. S. Lazarus, J. F. Hammerstone, and H. H. Schmitz, "Chocolate contains additional flavonoids not found in tea," *Lancet*, 1999, 354: 1825.
20. C. Tabak, I. C. Arts, H. A. Smit, D. Heederik, and D. Kromhout, "Chronic obstructive pulmonary disease and intake of catechins, flavonols, and flavones: the MORGEN Study," *Am J Respir Crit Care Med*, July 1, 2001, 164(1): 61–4.
21. K. H. van het Hof, H. S. de Boer, S. A. Wiseman, N. Lien, J. A. Westrate, and L. B. Tijburg, "Consumption of green or black tea does not increase resistance of low-density lipoprotein to oxidation in humans," *Am J Clin Nutr*, Nov. 1997, 66(5): 1125–32.

22. C. Sanbongi, N. Suzuki, and T. Sakane, "Polyphenols in chocolate, which have antioxidant activity, modulate immune functions in humans in vitro," *Cell Immunol,* 1997, 177(2): 129–36.

23. I. C. Arts; D. R. Jacobs, Jr.; L. J. Harnack; M. Gross; and A. R. Folsom; "Dietary catechins in relation to coronary heart disease death among postmenopausal women;" *Epidemiology;* Nov. 2001; 12(6): 668–75.

24. T. M. Haqqi, "Proceedings of the Nat. Academy of Sciences," 1999, 96: 4524–4529.

25. H. H. Lee, Y. Wuh, Y. C. Cuang et. al., "Epidemiologic characteristics and multiple risk factors of stomach cancer in Taiwan," *Anticancer Res,* 1990, 10: 875–81.

26. Zuo-Feng Zhang, *International Journal of Cancer,* 2001, 92: 600–604.

27. Y. Tsubono et al., "Green tea and the risk of gastric cancer in Japan," *N Engl J Med,* Mar 1, 2001, 344(9): 632–6.

28. Y. Hoshiyama et al., "A prospective study of stomach cancer death in relation to green tea consumption in Japan," *Br J Cancer,* Jul 29, 2002, 87(3): 309–13.

29. I. C. Arts, P. C. Hollman, E. J. Feskens, H. B. Bueno de Mesquita, and D. Kromhout, *Eur J Clin Nutr,* Feb 2001, 55(2): 76–81.

30. I. C. Arts, P. C. Hollman, H. B. Bueno De Mesquita, E. J. Feskens, and D. Kromhout, *Int J Cancer,* Apr 15, 2001, 92(2): 298–302.

31. J. L. Bushman, "Green Tea and Cancer in Humans: A Review of the Literature," *Nutr Cancer,* 1998, 31(3): 151–9.

32. M. Hirose, T. Hoshiya, Y. Mizoguchi, A. Nakamura, K. Akagi, and T. Shirai, "Green tea catechins enhance tumor development in the colon . . ." *Cancer,* Lett Jul 10, 2001, 168(1): 23–9.

33. T. J. Hartman, A. Joseph, J. A. Tangrea, P. Pietinen, P. N. Malila, M. Virtanen, P. R. Taylor, and D. Albanes, "Tea and Coffee Consumption and Risk of Colon and Rectal Cancer in Middle-Aged Finnish Men," *Nutrition and Cancer,* 1998, 31(1): 41–48.

34. C. H. Turner et al., "Fluoride treatment increased serum IGF-1, bone turnover, and bone mass, but not bone strength, in rabbits," *Calcif Tissue Int,* Jul 1997, 61(1): 77–83.

Soy

1 C. R. Sirtori, "Risks and benefits of soy phytoestrogens in cardiovascular diseases, cancer, climacteric symptoms and osteoporosis," *Drug Saf,* 2001, 24(9): 665–82.

2. H. Funahashi et al., "Seaweed prevents breast cancer?" *Jpn J Cancer Res,* May 2001, 92(5): 483–487.

3. Sally Fallon and Mary Enig, Ph.D., "Tragedy and Hype: The Third International Soy Symposium," *Nexus Magazine,* Volume 7, Number 3, April–May, 2000. (Based on the findings of Colin T. Campbell et al., *The Cornell Project in China.*)

4. C. Nagata, N. Takatsuka, Y. Kurisu, and H. Shimizu, "Decreased serum total choles-terol concentration is associated with high intake of soy products in Japanese men and women," *J Nutr,* Feb. 1998, 128(2): 209–213.

5. Sirtori.

6. Fallon and Enig.

7. Personal communication, Sally Fallon (www.westonaprice.org).

8. C. Dees, "Dietary estrogens stimulate human breast cells to enter the cell cycle," *Environmental Health Perspectives,* 1997, 105(Suppl. 3): 633–636.

9. Daniel M. Sheehan and Daniel R. Doerge, Letter to Dockets Management Branch (HFA-305), February 18, 1999.

10. L. Strauss et al., "Dietary phytoestrogens and their role in hormonally dependent disease," *Toxicol Lett,* Dec 28, 1998, 102–103: 349–354.

11. Third Meeting of the Open-ended Ad hoc Working Group on Biosafety of the UN-Convention on Biological Diversity, Montreal, October 13, 1997.

12. S. Carson, "The Shadow of Soy Or, How I Stopped Loving and Learned to Worry about the Bean," *The Pacific Sun*, Mill Valley, California, May 15, 2002. (Based on findings from: C. Irvine, et al. "The Potential Adverse Effects of Soybean Phytoestrogens in Infant Feeding," *New Zealand Medical Journal*, May 24, 1995.)

13. A. Cassidy, S. Bingham, and K. D. Setchell, "Biological effects of a diet of soy protein rich in isoflavones on the menstrual cycle of premenopausal women," *Am J Clin Nutr*, Sep 1994, 60(3): 333–340.

14. P. Fort, N. Moses, M. Fasano, T. Goldberg, and F. Lifshitz, "Breast and soy-formula feedings in early infancy and the prevalence of autoimmune thyroid disease in children," *J Am Coll Nutr*, Apr 1990, 9(2): 164–167.

15. P. Fort, R. Lanes, S. Dahlem, B. Recker, M. Weyman-Daum, M. Pugliese, and F. J. Lifshitz, "Breast feeding and insulin-dependent diabetes mellitus in children, *Am Coll Nutr*, 1986, 5(5): 439–441.

16. S. Yellayi et al., "The phytoestrogen genistein induces thymic and immune changes: a human health concern?" *Proc Natl Acad Sci*, May 28, 2002, 99(11): 7616–7621.

17. Press Release From Lehigh University, Department of Biochemical Sciences, Public release date: Oct 17, 2001.

18. Sheehan and Doerge.

19. Sirtori.

20. V. James. "The Committed on Toxicity in Foods and the Environment," *Wise Traditions*, Vol. 3, No. 4, Winter 2002, pp. 44–45.

21. www.soyonlineservice.co.nz.

22. Y. Ishisuki et al., "The effects on the thyroid gland of soybeans administered experimentally in healthy subjects," *Nippon Nibunpi Gawk Zasshi*, 1991, 67: 622–629.

23. *Ibid.*

24. E. Ashton and M. Ball, "Effects of soy as tofu vs. meat on lipoprotein concentrations," *Eur J Clin Nutr*, Jan 2000, 54(1): 14–19.

25. I. E. Liener, "Possible adverse effects of soybean anticarcinogens," *J Nutr*, Mar 1995, 125(3 Suppl): 744S–750S.

26. Robert Crayhon, *The Carnitine Miracle* (New York: Evans and Company, 1998).

27. Sally Fallon with Mary Enig, Ph.D., *Nourishing Traditions* (Washington, D.C.: New Trends Publishing, Inc., 1999, 2001).

28. J. Blankenship et al., "Lipoprotein (a) increased on vegan type diet and powdered soy milk," School of Public Health, Department of Medicine, Loma Linda University School of Medicine, Loma Linda, CA. Department of Medicine, Weimar Institute.

29. Ishisuki.

30. Nagata.

31. Haddow et al., "Maternal thyroid deficiency during pregnancy and subsequent neuropsychological development of the child," *N Engl J Med*, Aug 19, 1999, 341(8): 549–555.

32. Fallon and Enig.

33. C. Nagata et al., "Soy product intake and serum isoflavonoid and estradiol concentrations in relation to bone mineral density in postmenopausal Japanese women," *Osteoporos Int*, Mar 2002, 13(3): 200–4.

34. L. K. Massey, R. G. Palmer, and H. T. Horner, "Oxalate content of soybean seeds (Glycine max: Leguminosae), soyfoods, and other edible legumes," *J Agric Food Chem*, Sep 2001, 49(9): 4262–4266.

35. T. Hirayama, "A large scale cohort study on cancer risks by diet—with special reference to the risk reducing effects of green-yellow vegetable consumption," Princess Takamatsu Symposium (1985), 16: 41–53.

36. L. Coward et al., "Genistein, daidzein and their beta-glycoside conjugates: Antitumor isoflavones in soybean food from American and Asian diets," *J Agric Food Chem*, Nov 1993, 41(11): 1961–1967.
37. T. J. Key et al., "Soya foods and breast cancer risk: a prospective study in Hiroshima and Nagasaki, Japan," *Br J Cancer*, Dec 1999, 81(7): 1248–1256.
38. L. R. White et al., "Brain aging and midlife tofu consumption," *J Am Coll Nutr*, Apr 2000, 19(2): 242–255.

Cholesterol
1. Robert Crayhon, *Nutrition Made Simple* (New York: M. Evans, 1994).
2. Sally Fallon and Mary Enig, Ph.D., "It's the Beef," *Wise Traditions in Food, Farming and the Healing Arts*, Vol. 1, No. 1, Spring 2000, pp. 27–35.
3. J. Brunner and T. Bronisch, "Neurobiological correlates of suicidal behaviour," *Fortschritte der Neurologie-Psychiatrie*, Sep 1999, 67(9): 391–412.
4. L. F. Ellison and H. I. Morrison, "Low serum cholesterol concentration and risk of suicide,"*Epidemiology*, Mar 2001, 12(2): 168–172.
5. M. Sarchiapone, A. Roy, G. Camardese, and S. De Risio, "Further evidence for low serum cholesterol and suicidal behavior," *J Affect Discord*, Dec 1, 2000, 61(1-2): 69–71.
6. Sally Fallon with Mary Enig, Ph.D., *Nourishing Traditions* (Washington, D.C.: New Trends Publishing, 2001).
7. J. L. Richard et al., "Blood cholesterol and mortality," *Arch Mal Coeur Vaiss*, Oct 1992, 85 (Spec No 3): 11–19.
8. S. A. Missmer et al., "Meat and dairy food consumption and breast cancer: a pooled analysis of cohort studies," *Int J Epidemiol*, Feb 2002, 31(1): 78–85.
9. L. J. Vatten and O. P. Foss, "Total serum cholesterol and triglycerides and risk of breast cancer: a prospective study of 24,329 Norwegian women," *Cancer Res*, Apr 15, 1990, 50(8): 2341–2346.
10. Fallon and Enig, "It's the Beef."
11. S. B. Hulley, J. M. Walsh, and T. B. Newman, "Health policy on blood cholesterol. Time to change direction," *Circulation*, Sep 1992, 86(3): 1026–1029.
12. I. J. Schatz et al., "Cholesterol and all-cause mortality in elderly people from the Honolulu Heart Program: a cohort study," *Lancet*, Aug 4, 2001, 358(9279): 351–355.
13. Uffe Ravnskov, *The Cholesterol Myths* (Washington, D.C.: New Trends Publishing, 2000).
14. *Ibid.*
15. *Ibid.*
16. *Ibid.*
17. Mary Enig, *Know Your Fats: The Complete Primer for Understanding the Nutrition of Fats, Oils, and Cholesterol* (Maryland: Bethesda Press, 2000).
18. C. V. Felton et al., "Dietary Polyunsaturated Fatty Acids and Composition of Human Aortic Plaques," *Lancet*, 1994, 344: 1195.
19. R. Garrison and E. Somer, *The Nutrition Desk Reference* (New Canaan, CT: Keats Publishing, 1995).
20. A. S. Wells, N. W. Read, J. D. Laugharne, and N. S. Ahluwalia, "Alterations in mood after changing to a low-fat diet," *Br J Nutr*, Jan 1998, 79(1): 23–30.
21. Ravnskov.
22. Fallon and Enig, *Nourishing Traditions*.
23. *Ibid.*
24. W. Stillwell, T. Dallman, A. C. Dumaual, F. T. Crump, and L. J. Jenski, "Cholesterol versus alpha-tocopherol: effects on properties of bilayers made from heteroacid phosphatidylcholines," *Biochemistry*, Oct 15, 1996, 35(41): 13353–13362.

25. E. M. Cranton and J. P. Frackelton "Free Radical Pathology in Age-Associated Diseases: Treatment with EDTA Chelation, Nutrition and Antioxidants," *Journal of Holistic Medicine*, Spring/Summer 1984.

26. M. C. Vohl, T. A. Neville, R. Kumarathasan, S. Braschi, and D. L. Sparks, " A novel lecithin-cholesterol acyltransferase antioxidant activity prevents the formation of oxidized lipids during lipoprotein oxidation," *Biochemistry*, May 11, 1999, 38(19): 5976–5981.

27. Fallon and Enig, *Nourishing Traditions*.

28. *Ibid*.

29. *Ibid*. (W. Castelli, "Archives of Internal Medicine," Jul 1992, 152(7): 1371–1372.)

30. W. E. Kraus et al., "Effects of the amount and intensity of exercise on plasma lipoproteins," *N Engl J Med*, Nov 7, 2002, 347(19): 1483–1492.

31. C. B. Hollenbeck, "Dietary Fructose Effects on Lipoprotein Metabolism and Risk for Coronary Artery Disease," *American Journal of Clinical Nutrition*, 1993, 58(suppl): 800S–807S.

32. J. Hallfrisch et al., "The Effects of Fructose on Blood Lipid Levels," *American Journal of Clinical Nutrition*, 1983, 37(3): 740–748.

33 M. T. Shokravi et al., "Vitamin D inhibits angiogenesis in transgenic murine retinoblastoma," *Inv Oph*, 1995, 36: 83–87.

34. H. G. Ansleigh, "Beneficial effects of sun exposure on cancer mortality," *Prev Med*, 1993, 22: 132–140.

35. R. Hobday, *The Healing Sun*. (Forres, UK: Findhorn Press, 1999).

36. K. S. McCully, *The Homocysteine Revolution* (New Canaan, CT: Keats Publishing, Inc., 1997).

37. P. Ridker, J. E. Manson, J. E. Buring et al., "Homocysteine and risk of cardiovascular disease among postmenopausal women," *JAMA*, 1999, 281: 1817–1821.

38. M. J. Stampfer, R. Malinow, W. C. Willett et al., "A prospective study of plasma homocysteine and risk of myocardial infarction in US physicians," *JAMA*, 1992, 268:877–881.

39. L. E. Brattstrom, B. L. Hultberg, and J. E. Hardebo, "Folic acid responsive postmenopausal homocysteinemia," *Metabolism*, 1985, 34: 1073–1077.

40. R. Clarke, D. Smith, and K. A. Jobst et al., "Folate, vitamin B12, and serum total homocysteine levels in confirmed Alzheimer disease," *Arch Neurol*, 1998, 55: 1449–1455.

41. J. M. Schwarz, P. Linfoot, D. Dare, and K. Aghajanian, "Hepatic de novo lipogenesis in normoinsulinemic subjects consuming high-fat, low-carbohydrate and low-fat, high-carbohydrate isoenergetic diets," *Am J Clin Nutr*, Jan 2003, 77(1): 43–50.

42. S. Gallisti et al., "Insulin is an independent correlate of plasma homocysteine levels in obese children and adolescents," *Diabetes Care*, Sep 2000, 23(9): 1348–1352.

43. J. Chan, S. F. Knutsen, G. G. Blix, J. W. Lee, and G. E. Fraser, "Water, other fluids, and fatal coronary heart disease: the Adventist Health Study," *Am J Epidemiol*, May 1, 2002, 155(9): 827–833.

44. Enig, *Know Your Fats*.

45. K. C. Hayes, "Saturated fats and blood lipids: new slant on an old story," *Can J Cardiol*, Oct 1995,11(Suppl G): 39G–46G.

46. H. L. Newbold, "Reducing the serum cholesterol level with a diet high in animal fat," *South Med J*, Jan 1988, 81(1): 61–63.

47. W. Castelli, "Concerning the possibility of a nut . . ." *Archives of Internal Medicine*, July 1992, 152(7), 1371–1372.

48. Udo Erasmus, *Fats That Heal—Fats That Kill* (Burnaby, B.C., Canada: Alive Books, 1993).

49. Robert Crayhon, *The Carnitine Miracle* (New York: M. Evans, 1998).

50. A. Schatzkin, E. Lanza, D. Corle et al., "The Polyp Prevention Trial Study Group. Lack of Effect of a Low-Fat, High-Fiber Diet on the Recurrence of Colorectal Adenomas," *N Eng J of Med*, 2000, 342: 1149–1155.

51. A. Ascherio et. al. "Dietary fat and risk of coronary heart disease in men: cohort follow up study in the United States," *British Medical Journal*, Jul 13, 1996, 313(7049): 84–90.

52. B. Koletzko and J. Muller, "Cis- and Trans-Isomeric Fatty Acids in Plasma Lipids of Newborn Infants and Their Mothers," *Biology of the Neonate*, 1990, 57: 172–178.

53. G.V. Mann, "Metabolic Consequences of Dietary Trans Fatty Acids," *The Lancet*, 1994, 343: 1268–1271.

54. W. C.Willett et al., "Intake of Trans Fatty Acids and Risk of Coronary Heart Disease Among Women," *Lancet*, 1993, 341: 581–585.

55. Enig, *Know Your Fats*.

56. T. Dunder, L. Kiukka, J. Turtinen, L. Rasanen, and M. Uhari, "Diet, serum fatty acids, and atopic diseases in childhood," *Allergy*, May 2001, 56(5): 425–428.

57. Mary G. Enig, Ph.D., and Sally Fallon, "The Oiling of America," first published in *Nexus Magazine*, Dec 1998–Jan 1999 and Feb 1999–Mar 1999.

58. Crayhon, *The Carnitine Miracle*.

59. G. L. Blackburn, G. Kater, E. A. Mascioli, M. Kowalchuk, V. K. Babayan, and B. R. Bistrian, " A re-evaluation of coconut oil's effect on serum cholesterol and atherogenesis," *The Journal of the Philippine Medical Association*, 1989, 65: 144–152.

60. *Nutrition Action Health Letter*, Center for Science in the Public Interest, Washington, D.C., Nov 1990.

61. www.nas.edu.

62. N. M. deRoos, M. L. Bots, and M. B. Katan, "Replacement of dietary saturated fatty acids by trans fatty acids lowers serum HDL cholesterol and impairs endothlial function in healthy men and women," *Arterioscler Thromb Vasc Biol,* Jul 2001, 21(7): 1233–1237.

63. *Nutrition Action Health Letter*, Oct 1990.

64. *Ibid*.

65. L. Kohlmeier et al., "Stores of Trans Fatty Acids and Breast Cancer Risk, "*Am J Clin Nutr*, 1995, 61:896, A25.

66. Willett.

67. Enig, *Know Your Fats*.

68. P. Khosla and K. C. Hayes, "Dietary trans-monounsaturated fatty acids negatively impact plasma lipids in humans: critical review of the evidence," *J Am Coll Nutr*, Aug 1996, 15(4): 321–322.

69. Fallon and Enig, *Nourishing Traditions*.

70. Ravnskov.

Conjugated Linoleic Acid

1. S.Visonneau et al., "Conjugated linoleic acid suppresses the growth of human breast adenocarcinoma cells in SCID mice," *Anticancer Research* (Greece), 1997, 17(2 A): 969–973.

2. P.W. Parodi, "Cows' milk fat components as potential anticarcinogenic agents," *Journal of Nutrition,* 1997, 127(6): 1055–1060.

3. T. D. Shultz, B. P. Chew, W. R. Seaman, and L. O. Luedecke, "Inhibitory effect of conjugated dienoic derivatives of linoleic acid and beta-carotene on the in vitro growth of human cancer cells," *Cancer Lett.*, 1992, 63(2): 125–133.

4. C. Ip, J. A. Scimeca, and H. J. Thompson, "Conjugated linoleic acid: A powerful anticarcinogen from animal fat sources," *Cancer,* 1994, 74(3): 1050–1054.

5. C. Ip, M. Singh, H. J. Thompson, and J. A. Scimeca, "Conjugated linoleic acid suppresses mammary carcinogenesis and proliferative activity of the mammary gland in the rat," *Cancer Res*, Mar 1, 1994, 54(5): 1212–1215.
6. H. M. Roche, E. Noone, A. Nugent, and M. J. Gibney, "Conjugated linoleic acid: a novel therapeutic nutrient," *Nutr. Res. Rev*, 2001, 14:173–187.
7. T. D. Shultz, B. P. Chew, W. R. Seaman, and L. O. Luedecke, "Inhibitory effect of conjugated dienoic derivatives of linoleic acid and beta-carotene on the in vitro growth of human cancer cells," *Cancer Lett*, Apr 15, 1992, 63(2): 125–133.
8. C. Steinhart, "Conjugated Linoleic Acid—The Good News about Animal Fat," *J. Chem. Educ*, 1996, vol.73, no.12, p. A302.
9. R. J. Nicolosi et al., "Dietary conjugated linoleic acid reduces plasma lipoproteins and early aortic atherosclerosis in hypercholesterolemic hamsters," *Artery*, 1997, 22(5): 266–277.
10. K. N. Lee, D. Kritchevsky, and M. W. Pariza, "Conjugated linoleic acid and atherosclerosis in rabbits," *Atherosclerosis*, 1994, 108(1): 19–25.
11. S. Reiner, "CLA: Does Fat Have a Silver Lining?" *Health Priorities*, Vol. 8, Number 4, 1996: 44–47 (www.acsh.org/publications/priorities/0804/cla.html).
12. I. Greenwell, "Lose the Fat—Keep the Muscle," *Life Extension Magazine*, April 1999: 14–18.
13. R. L. Atkinson, "Conjugated linoleic acid for altering body composition and treating obesity," in *Advances in Conjugated Linoleic Acid Research*, eds. M. P. Yurawecz, M. M. Mossoba, J. K. G. Kramer, M. W. Pariza, and G. J. Nelson (Champaign, IL: AOCS Press, 1999) Vol. 1, pp. 348–353.
14. H. Blankson, J. A. Stakkestad, H. Fagertun et al., "Conjugated linoleic acid reduces body fat mass in overweight and obese humans," *J Nutr*, 2000, 130: 2943–2948.
15. A. Smedman and B. Vessby, "Conjugated linoleic acid supplementation in humans—metabolic effects," *Lipids*, Aug 2001, 36(8): 773–781.
16. M. A. Belury, A. Mahon, and S. Banni, "The conjugated linoleic acid (CLA) isomer, t10c12-CLA, is inversely associated with changes in body weight and serum leptin in subjects with type 2 diabetes mellitus," *J Nutr*, Jan 2003, 133(1): 257S–260S.
17. C. Ip et al., "The efficacy of conjugated linoleic acid in mammary cancer prevention is independent of the level or type of fat in the diet," *Carcinogenesis*, 1996, 17(5): 1045–1050.
18. T. R. Dhiman, G. R. Anand, L. D. Satter et al., "Conjugated linoleic acid content of milk from cows fed different diets," *Journal of Dairy Science*, 1996, 79(Supplement 1): 137.
19. Reiner.
20. Z. Balogh, J. I. Gray, E. A. Gomaa, A. M. Booren, "Formation and inhibition of heterocyclic aromatic amines in fried ground beef patties," *Food Chem Toxicol*, May 2000, 38(5): 395–401.
21. J. Raloff, "Well-Done Research," *Science News Online—The Weekly Newsmagazine of Science,* Vol. 155, No. 17, April 24, 1999, www.sciencenews.org/sn_arc9914_24_99/bob1.htm.
22. C. P. Salmon et al., "Effects of marinating on heterocyclic amine carcinogen formation in grilled chicken," *Food Chem Toxicol*, 1997, 35: 433–441.
23. L. Zimmerman, "Simple Steps to Healthier Grilling," *Consumer Update,* Univ. of Missouri, Lincoln Universit, August 1997.
24. P. V. Nerurkar, L. Le Marchand, and R. V. Cooney, "Effects of marinating with Asian marinades or western barbecue sauce on PhIP and MeIQx formation in barbecued beef," *Nutr Cancer*, 1999, 34(2): 147–152.
25. R. F. Schmid, *Traditional Foods Are Your Best Medicine* (New York: Ballantine Books, 1978).

26. J. B. Russel, F. Diez-Gonzalez, and G. N. Jarvis, "Potential effect of cattle diets on the transmission of pathogenic *Escherichia coli* to humans," *Microbes Infect*, Jan 2000, 2(1): 45–53.

27. R. M. Williams, "Environmental Issues: What's Milk Got?" *Townsend Letter for Doctors and Patients*, Oct 2002, www.townsendletter.com/oct_2002/milk1002.htm.

28. Y. Huang, L. Luedecke, and T. Shultz, "Effect of cheddar cheese consumption on plasma conjugated linoleic acid concentrations in men," *Nutr Res*, 1994, 14(3): 373–386.

29. J. Raloff, "Cheese source of dietary anticancer agent," *Science News*, Feb.11, 1989, 135: 87.

30. P. Brougnoux, F. Lavillonniere, and E. Riboli, "Inverse relationship between CLA in adipose breast tissue and risk of breast cancer. A case-control study in France," *Inform*, 1999, 1(5): s43.

31. P. Knekt et al., "Intake of dairy products and the risk of breast cancer," *Br J Cancer*, Mar 1996, 73(5): 687–691.

32. A. Hjartaker, P. Laake, and E. Lund, "Childhood and adult milk consumption and risk of premenopausal breast cancer," *Int J Cancer*, Sep 15, 2001, 93(6): 888–893.

33. P. van't Veer et al., "Consumption of fermented milk products and breast cancer: a case-control study in The Netherlands," *Cancer Res*, Jul 15, 1989, 49(14): 4020–4023.

34. A. Aro et al., "Inverse association between dietary and serum conjugated linoleic acid and risk of breast cancer in postmenopausal women," *Nutr Cancer*, 2000, 38(2): 151–157.

35. B. Gottlieb, *Alternative Cures* (Emmaus, PA: Rodale Press, 2000).

36. S. Basu, U. Riserus, A. Turpeinen, and B. Vessby, "Conjugated linoleic acid induces lipid peroxidation in men with abdominal obesity," *Clin Sci*, Dec 2000, 99 (6): 511–516.

Fluoridation

1. R. P. Ellwood and D. O'Mullane, "The association between developmental enamel defects and caries in populations with and without fluoride in their drinking water," *J Public Health Dent*, 1996, 56(2): 76–80.

2. M. T. Alarcon-Herrera et al., "Well water fluoride, dental fluorosis and bone fractures in the Guadiana Valley of Mexico," *Fluoride*, 2001, 34: 139–150.

3. P. Hauser, "Attention deficit-hyperactivity disorder in people with generalized resistance to thyroid hormone," *N Engl J Med*, Apr 8, 1993, 328(14): 997–1001.

4. R. D. Masters and M. Coplan, "Water treatment with Silicofluorides and Lead Toxicity," *International Journal of Environmental Studies*, September, 1989, pp. 435–449.

5. H. C. Moolenburgh, "Fluoridation in Holland—injuries to health—personal communication," *Pak Dent Rev*, Jan–Apr 1979, 27(1-2): 24–26.

6. J. Luke, "Fluoride deposition in the aged human pineal gland," *Caries Res*, Mar–Apr 2001, 35(2): 125–128.

7. J. R. Lee, M.D., et al., *What Your Doctor May Not Tell You About Breast Cancer* (Hopkins, Virginia: Warner Books, 2002).

8. P. J. Mullenix, P. K. Denbesten, and A. Schunior, "Neurotoxicity of sodium fluoride in rats," *Neurotoxicology and Teratology*, 1995, 17(2): 169–177.

9. T. Schettler, J. Stein, F. Reich, and M. Valenti, "In Harm's Way: Toxic Threats to Child Development," *Greater Boston Physicians for Social Responsibility*, May 2000, http://psr.igc.org/ihw.htm.

10. B. L. Douglas et al., "Impact of water fluoridation on dental practice and dental manpower," *J Am Dent Assoc*, Feb 1972, 84(2): 355–367.

11. State of California, Department of Health Services, Medical Statistics Section for recipients qualified for Medi-Cal dental treatments for 1994 and 1995.

12. J. W. Hirzy, Ph.D., "Scientific Integrity in a Regulatory Context—An Elusive Ideal at EPA," *Second Look*, July 9, 2002, www.slweb.org.
13. *Review of Fluoride Benefits and Risks*, U.S. Department of Health and Human Services, 1991, p. 45.
14. C. Savas, M. Cetin, M. Akdogan, and N. Heybeli, "Endemic fluorosis in Turkish patients: relationship with knee osteoarthritis," *Rheumatol Int*, Sep 2001, 21 (1): 30–35.
15. L. Krook and R. R. Minor, "Fluoride and Alkaline Phosphatase," *Fluoride* 1198 (New York, Cornell University, 1998) 31: 177–182.
16. P. Connett, *Fluoride: A Statement of Concern* (NY: St. Lawrence University, Nov 1999).
17. J. Colquhoun, Chief Dental Officer, NZ, International Symposium on Fluoridation (Porte Alegre, Brazil, September 1988).
18. C. Bryson and J. Griffiths, "Fluoride, Teeth and the Atomic Bomb," *Waste Not*, September 1997, pp. 1–8.
19. X. S. Li, J. L. Zhi, and R. O. Gao, "Effect of fluoride exposure on intelligence in children," *Fluoride* 28 (1995), pp. 189–192.
20. L. B. Zhao, G. H. Liang, D. N. Zhang, and X. R. Wu, "Effect of high fluoride water supply on children's intelligence," *Fluoride* (1996), 29: 190–192.
21. Proceedings, *City of Orville vs. Public Utilities Commission of the State of California* (Orville, CA, October 20-21, 1955).
22. D. Edell, *Eat, Drink and Be Merry* (New York: Harper Collins, 1999).
23. A. Weil, *8 Weeks to Optimal Health*. (New York: Knopf, 1997).
24. *Why EPA's Headquarters Union of Scientists Opposes Fluoridation*, prepared on behalf of the National Treasury Employees Union, Chapter 280, by Chapter Senior Vice-President J. William Hirzy, Ph.D.
25. P. D. Cohn, "A brief report on the association of drinking water fluoridation and the incidence of osteosarcoma among young males" (New Jersey Department of Health, 1992).
26. J. A. Varner, K. F. Jensen, W. Horvath, and R. L. Isaacson, "Chronic administration of aluminum-fluoride or sodium-fluoride to rats in drinking water: alterations in neuronal and cerebrovascular integrity," *Brain Res*, Feb 16, 1998, 784(1-2): 284–298.
27. A. Strunecka and J. Patocka, "Reassessment of the role of aluminum in the development of Alzheimer's disease," *Cesk Fysiol*, Feb 1999, 48(1): 9–15.
28. Andreas Schuld, http://www.bruha.com/fluoride/.
29. J. Yiamouyiannis, *Fluoride, The Aging Factor* (Delaware, OH: Health Action Press, 1986).
30. Trustees of Dartmouth College. "Dartmouth Researcher Warns of Chemicals Added to Drinking Water" (March 15, 2001) www.dartmouth.edu/~news.
31. Affidavit of Albert Schatz, Ph.D., in Support of Motion for Summary Judgment (Circuit Court Fond Du Lac County, Wisconsin, Case No. 92 CV 579, 1993).
32. J. D. Featherstone, "The science and practice of caries prevention," *J Am Dent Assoc*, Jul 2000, 131(7): 887–899.
33. Barry Forbes, "Prominent researcher apologizes for pushing fluoride," *The Tribune* (Mesa, AZ), Sunday, December 5, 1999, http://pwgazette.com/hardylimeback.htm.

Aspartame

1. Betty Martini, original Internet article: http://nancymarkle.com/betty/betty.html.
2. W. C. Monte, "Aspartame: Methanol and the Public Health," *Journal of Applied Nutrition*, 1984, 36 (1): 42–53.
3. P. R. Camfield, C. S. Camfield, J. M. Dooley et al., "Aspartame exacerbates eeg spike wave discharge in children with generalized absence epilepsy, a double-blind controlled study," *Neurology*, 1992, 42: 1000–1003.
4. L. J. Elsas, II, M.D.; Director, Division of Medical Genetics; Professor of Pediatrics, Emory University School of Medicine. Statement before the Committee of Labor

and Human Resources on the subject "Nutrasweet: Health and safety concerns," November 3, 1987.

5. Joseph Mercola, http://www.mercola.com/article/aspartame/.

6. J. W. Olney, "Aspartame as a sweetener," *New Engl J Med*, 1975, 2(2)23: 1244–1245.

7. H. J. Roberts, "Aspartame effects during pregnancy and childhood" (letter), *Latitudes*, 1997, 3(No. 1): 3.

8. R. G. Walton, R. Hudak, and R. J. Green-Waite, "Adverse reactions to aspartame; Double-blind challenge in patients from a vulnerable population," *Biol Psychiatry*, 1993, 34(1-2): 13–17.

9. H. J. Roberts, "Neurologic psychiatric and behavioral reactions to aspartame in 505 aspartame reactors," eds. Wurtman and Ritter-Walker, *Dietary Phenylalanine and Brain Function* (Boston: Birkhauser, 1988), pp. 373–376.

10. R. L. Blaylock, *Excitotoxins: The Taste That Kills* (Santa Fe, New Mexico: Health Press, 1994).

11. J. W. Olney, N. B. Farber, E. Spitznagel, and L. Robins, "Increasing brain tumor rates: Is there a link to aspartame?" *J Neuropathol Exp Neurol*, 1996, 55(11): 1115–1123.

12. H. J. Roberts, *Aspartame (NutraSweet). Is it Safe?* (Philadelphia, PA: The Charles Press, 1992).

13. "In response to allegations by the Community Nutrition Institute (CNI) and Dr. John Olney regarding aspartame," Joint Statement of the Calorie Control Council, National Food Processors Association, Grocery Manufacturers of America, National Soft Drink Association.

14. Mercola.

15. U.S. Department of Health and Human Services, Report on All Adverse Reactions in the Adverse Reaction Monitoring System, February 25 and 28, 1994.

16. "Aspartame Adverse Reaction Reports Down in 1994 From 1985 Peak: FDA," *Food Chemical News*, June 12, 1995, p. 27.

17. U.S. Air Force. "Aspartame Alert," *Flying Safety*, May 1992, 48 (5): 20–21.

18. R. G. Walton, "Seizure and mania after high intake of aspartame," *Psychosomatics*, 1986, 27: 218–220.

19. R. J. Wurtmann, "Aspartame: Possible effects on seizure susceptibility," *Lancet*, 1985, 2(8463): 1060.

20. H. J. Roberts, *Aspartame Disease: An Ignored Epidemic* (West Palm Beach, FL: Sunshine Sentinel Press, Inc., 2001).

21. H. J. Roberts, "Aspartame effects . . ." (letter).

22. Elsas.

23. J. W. Olney, "Brain damage in infant mice following oral intake of glutamate, aspartate or cysteine," *Nature*, 1970, 227: 609–610.

24. J. W. Olney, "Brain damage in mice from voluntary ingestion of glutamate and aspartate," *Neurobehav Toxicol Teratol*, 1980, 2: 125–129.

25. D. C. Rice, "Parallels between attention deficit hyperactivity disorder and behavioral deficits produced by neurotoxic exposure in monkeys," *Environ Health Perspect*, Jun 2000, 108(Suppl 3): 405–408.

26. George Schwartz. "Correcting Internet Myths About NutraSweet," Letter to Team Nutrasweet Monsanto, February 2, 1999.

27. J. D. Smith et al., "Relief of Fibromyalgia Symptoms Following Discontinuation of Dietary Excitotoxins," *The Annals of Pharmacotherapy*, June 2001, Vol. 35, pp. 702–706.

28. D. R. Johns, "Migraine provoked by aspartame," *New Engl J Med*, 1986, 315(7): 456.

29. R. B. Lipton et al., "Aspartame as a dietary trigger of headache," *Headache*, Feb 1989, 29(2): 90–92.

30. H. J. Roberts, Director, Palm Beach Institute for Medical Research, "Aspartame (Nutrasweet) Addiction," *Townsend Letter for Doctors*, Jan. 2000, pp. 52–57.

31. M. G. Tordoff and A. M. Allera, "Oral stimulation with aspartame increases hunger," *Physiol Behav*, Mar 1990, 47(3): 555–559.
32. R. M. Black, L. A. Leiter, and G. H. Anderson, "Consuming aspartame with and without taste: differential effects on appetite and food intake of young adults," *Physiol Behav*, Mar 1993, 53(3): 459–466.
33. Joseph Mercola. "Aspartame—History of Fraud and Deception," www.mercola.com/article/aspartame/fraud.htm.
34. M. N. Stoddard, *The Deadly Deception* (Dallas, TX: Odenwald Books, 1998).
35. Adrian Gross. Statement from Dr. Andrian Gross, Former FDA Investigator and Scientist, "Aspartame Safety Act" (Congressional Record, Vol. 131, No. 106, August 1, 1985).
36. U.S. Food and Drug Administration, Searle Investigation Task Force chaired by Carlton Sharp. "Final report of Investigation of G. D. Searle Company" (March 24, 1976).
37. E. Millstone, "Sweet and sour: The unanswered questions about aspartame," *The Ecologist*, 1994, 24(2): 71–74.
38. Gregory Gordon, "Nutrasweet Approval Marred by Controvers," www.dorway.com/upipaper.txt.
39. "Artificial Sweeteners: How safe?" (2001), http://worldwidescam.com/fdacoll.htm.
40. R. G. Walton, "Survey of Aspartame Studies: Correlation of Outcome and Funding Sources" (date?), Northeastern Ohio University's College of Medicine.
41. C. Trocho, R. Pardo, I. Rafecas, J. Virgili, X. Remesar, J. A. Fernandez-Lopez, and M. Alemany, "Formaldehyde derived from dietary aspartame binds to tissue components in vivo," *Life Sci*, 1998, 63(5): 337–349.
42. Bryant Holman, http://presidiotex.com/aspartame/Facts/PR/pr.html.

Osteoporosis

1. S. Sellman, "Osteoporosis—The Bones of Contention," *Nexus Magazine* (Oct-Nov 1998), Vol.5, No.6: 21–26.
2. M. Iki et al., "Bone mineral density of the spine, hip and distal forearm in representative samples of the Japanese female population: Japanese Population-Based Osteoporosis (JPOS) Study," *Osteoporos Int*, 2001, 12(7): 529–537.
3. P. D. Ross et al., "A comparison of hip fracture incidence among native Japanese, Japanese Americans, and American Caucasians," *Am J Epidemiol*, Apr 15, 1991, 133(8): 801–809.
4. H. Norimatsu, S. Mori, T. Uesato, T. Yoshikawa, and N. Katsuyama, "Bone mineral density of the spine and proximal femur in normal and osteoporotic subjects in Japan," *Bone Miner*, Jan 1989, 5(2): 213–222.
5. G. A. Colditz, "Relationships between estrogen levels, use of hormone replacement therapy and breast cancer," *J. NCI*, 1998, 90(11): 814–823.
6. G. A. Colditz et. al,. "The use of estrogens and progestins and the risk of breast cancer in postmenopausal women," *N Engl J Med*, Jun 15, 1995, 332(24): 1589–1593.
7. A. R. Gaby, *Preventing and Reversing Osteoporosis* (Rocklin, CA: Prima Publishing, 1994).
8. J. R. Lee, M.D., *What Your Doctor May Not Tell You About Menopause: The Breakthrough Book on Natural Progesterone* (Hopkins, Virginia: Warner Books, 1996).
9. A. H. Follingstad, "Estriol, the forgotten estrogen?" *JAMA*, Jan 2, 1978, 239(1): 29–30.
10. P. Alexandersen, A. Toussaint, C. Christiansen et al., "Ipriflavone in the treatment of postmenopausal osteoporosis: a randomized controlled trial," *JAMA*, 2001, 285:1482–1488.
11. Robert Crayhon, *Nutrition Made Simple* (New York: M. Evans and Co., 1994).

12. Sellman.
13. R. Bileckot, M. Audran, C. Masson, H. Ntsiba, P. Simon, and J. C. Renier, "Bone density in 20 black African young adults of the Bantu race is identical to that in subjects of white race," *Rev Rhum Mal Osteoartic*, Nov 30, 1991, 58(11): 787–789.
14. Sally Fallon with Mary Enig, Ph.D., *Nourishing Traditions* (Washington, D.C.: New Trends Publishing, Inc., 1999, 2001).
15. G. E. Abraham and H. Grewal, "A total dietary program emphasizing magnesium instead of calcium. Effect on the mineral density of calcaneous bone in postmenopausal women on hormonal therapy," *J Reprod Med*, May 1990, 35(5): 503–507.
16. A. L. Gittleman, *Your Body Knows Best* (New York: Pocket Books, 1996), www.fatflush.com.
17. G. E. Abraham et. al., "The Importance of Magnesium in the Management of Primary Postmenopausal Osteoporosis," *Journal of Nutritional Medicine*, 1991, 2: 165–178.
18. M. Kaneki et al., "Japanese fermented soybean food as the major determinant of the large geographic difference in circulating levels of vitamin K2: possible implications for hip-fracture risk," *Nutrition*, Apr 2001, 17(4): 315–321.
19. C. Nagata et al., "Soy product intake and serum isoflavonoid and estradiol concentrations in relation to bone mineral density in postmenopausal Japanese women," *Osteoporos Int*, Mar 2002, 13(3): 200–204.
20. H. Melhus et al. "Excessive dietary intake of vitamin A is associated with reduced bone mineral density and increased risk for hip fracture," *Ann Intern Med*, Nov 15, 1998, 129(10): 770–778.
21. S. J. Whiting and B. Lemke, "Excess retinol intake may explain the high incidence of osteoporosis in northern Europe," *Nutr Rev*, Jun 1999, 57(6): 192–195.
22. D. Rucker et al., (Departments of Medical Science, Medicine and Community Health Sciences, University of Calgary), "Vitamin D insufficiency in a population of healthy western Canadians," *CMAJ*, June 4, 2002, 166(12):1517–1424.
23. Crayhon.
24. P. D. Ross and C. Huang, "Hip fracture incidence among Caucasians in Hawaii is similar to Japanese. A population-based study." *Aging* (Milano), Oct 2000, 12(5): 356–359.
25. W. B. Grant, "An estimate of premature cancer mortality in the U.S. due to inadequate doses of solar ultraviolet-B radiation," *Cancer*, Mar 15, 2002, 94(6): 1867–1875.
26. J. P. Bonjour, M. A. Schurch, and R. Rizzoli, "Nutritional aspects of hip fractures," *Bone*, Mar 1996, 18(3 Suppl): 139S–144S.
27. J. P. Bonjour et al., "Proteins and bone health," *Pathol Biol* (Paris), Jan 1997, 45(1): 57–59.
28. R. G. Munger, J. R. Cerhan, and B. C. Chiu, "Prospective study of dietary protein intake and risk of hip fracture in postmenopausal women," *Am J Clin Nutr*, Jan 1999, 69(1): 147–152.
29. D. Teegarden et al., "Previous milk consumption is associated with greater bone density in young women," *Am J Clin Nutr*, May 1999, 69(5): 1014–1017.
30. S. I. Barr, J. C. Prior, K. C. Janelle, and B. C. Lentle, "Spinal bone mineral density in premenopausal vegetarian and nonvegetarian women: cross-sectional and prospective comparisons," *J Am Diet Assoc*, Jul 1998, 98(7): 760–765.
31. J. F. Chiu et al., "Long-term vegetarian diet and bone mineral density in postmenopausal Taiwanese women," *Calcif Tissue Int*, Mar 1997, 60(3): 245–249.
32. Teegarden.
33. J-F. Z. X-H. Hu, J-B. Jia et al., "Dietary calcium and bone density among middle-aged and elderly women in China," *Am J Clin Nutr*, 1993, 58: 219–227.

34. B. Dawson-Hughes and S. S. Harris, "Calcium intake influences the association of protein intake with rates of bone loss in elderly men and women," *Am J Clin Nutr,* Apr 2002, 75(4): 773–779.

35. D. Feskanich, W. C. Willett, M. J. Stampfer, and G. A. Colditz, "Protein consumption and bone fractures in women," *Am J Epidemiol,* Mar 1, 1996, 143(5): 472–479.

36. D. Feskanich, W. C. Willett, and G. A. Colditz, "Calcium, vitamin D, milk consumption, and hip fractures in postmenopausal women," *Am J Clin Nutr,* Feb 2003, 77(2): 504–511.

37. F. P. Cappuccio, R. Kalaitzidis, S. Duneclift, and J. B. Eastwood, "Unravelling the links between calcium excretion, salt intake, hypertension, kidney stones and bone metabolism," *J Nephrol,* May–Jun 2000, 13(3): 169–177.

38. Crayhon.

39. Y. Beyene and M. C. Martin, "Menopausal experiences and bone density of Mayan women in Yucatan, Mexico," *Am J Human Biol,* Jul–Aug 2001, 13(4): 505–511.

40. M. C. Martin, J. E. Block, S. D. Sanchez, C. D. Arnaud, and Y. Beyene, "Menopause without symptoms: the endocrinology of menopause among rural Mayan Indians," *Am J Obstet Gynecol,* Jun 1993, 168(6 Pt 1): 1839–1843.

41. S. Brown, Ph.D., *Better Bones, Better Body* (New Canaan, CT: Keats Publishing, 1996).

42. M. C. Kruger et al., "Calcium, gamma-linolenic acid and eicosapentaenoic acid supplementation in senile osteoporosis," *Aging,* Oct 1998, 10(5): 385–394.

43. B. A. Watkins, J. J. Turek, M. F. Seifert, and H. Xu, *Importance of Vitamin E in bone formation and in chondrocyte function,* (Indianapolis, IN: American Oil Chemists Society, 1996).

Bovine Growth Hormone

1. P. Montague, "Breast Cancer, rBGH and Milk," *Rachel's Environment & Health Weekly* #593, Environmental Research Foundation, May 8, 1998, http://www.monitor.net/rachel/.

2. P. Montague, "Milk, rBGH, and Cancer," *Rachel's Environmental and Health Weekly* #593, Apr. 9, 1998.

3. S. S. Epstein and O. Hardin, "Confidential Monsanto Research Files Dispute Many BGH Safety Claims," *The Milkweed,* 1990, Vol. 128, pgs. 3–6. Discusses P. J. Eppard and others, "Toxicity Of CP115099 In A Prolonged Release System In Lactating Cows." REPORT MSL 6345 (St.Louis, Mo.: Monsanto Agricultural Co., 1987). (As cited in *Rachel's Environmental and Health Weekly* #383, Mar 31, 1994.)

4. P. Montague, "Breast Cancer . . ."

5. C. G. Prosser, I. R. Fleet, and A. N. Corps, "Increased secretion of insulin-like growth factor 1 into milk of cows treated with recombinantly derived bovine growth hormone," *J Dairy Res,* Feb 1989, 56(1): 17–26.

6. S. E. Hankinson et. al., "Circulating concentrations of insulin-like growth factor I and risk of breast cancer," *Lancet,* May 9, 1998, 351(9113): 1393–1396.

7. J. M. Chan et al. "Plasma Insulin-Like Growth Factor-I and Prostate Cancer Risk: A Prospective Study," *Science,* Jan 23, 1998, 279: 563–566.

8. C. S. Mantzoros et al., "Insulin-like growth factor 1 in relation to prostate cancer and benign prostatic hyperplasia," *British Journal of Cancer,* 1997, 76(9): 1115-1118.

9. R. Torrisi, "Time course of ferretinide-induced modulation of circulating insulin-like growth factor (IGF)-i, IGF-II and IGFBP-3 in a bladder cancer chemoprevention trial," *J Cancer,* Aug 15, 2000, 87(4): 601–605.

10. C. H. Turner et al., "Fluoride treatment increased serum IGF-1, bone turnover, and bone mass, but not bone strength, in rabbits. *Calcif Tissue Int,* Oct 1997, 61(4): 349.

11. http://www2.okstate.edu/pio/soygroup2.html.

12. G. D. Smith, D. Gunnell, and J. Holly, "Cancer and insulin-like growth factor-1. A potential mechanism linking the environment with cancer risks," *BMJ*, Oct 7, 2000, 321(7265): 847–848.
13. Michael Hansen, "Living on Earth," transcript of radio interview (December 18, 1998).
14. S. S. Epstein, "Unlabeled milk from cows treated with biosynthetic growth hormones: a case of regulatory abdication," *Int J Health Servi*, 1996, 26(1): 173–185.
15. S. S. Epstein, "Potential public health hazards of biosynthetic milk hormones," *International Journal of Health Services*, 1990, Vol. 20, No. 1, pp. 73–84.
16. P. Montague, "How Monsanto 'Listens' to Other Opinions," *The Ecologist*, September/October 1998, p. 299.
17. B. Duplisea and L. Sharratt, "BGH Background" (Sierra Club of Canada, September 14, 1998), http://www.sierraclub.ca/national/genetic/bghback.htm.
18. *Ibid.*
19. *Ibid.*
20. S. Chopra et. al., "Gaps Analysis" Report, rBST Internal Review Team, rBST (Nutrilac), April 21, 1998.
21. L. Eggertson, "Expert worked for drug firm," *Toronto Star*, September 21, 1998, p. A2.
22. P. Montague, "Milk Controversy Spills into Canada," *Rachel's Environmental Health Weekly* #621, Oct. 22, 1998, http://www.greens.org/s-r/18/18-08.html.
23. P. Montague, "Milk, rBHG . . . "
24. "Reporters Win Lawsuit to Thwart Fox-TV Cover-Up," BGH Bulletin, 2000. http://www.foxbghsuit.com/
25. P. Montague, "Milk, rBHG . . . "
26. Michelle Thom, "Food Safety Week," Institute for Agriculture and Trade Policy (Feb. 25, 1994), www.sare.org/htdocs/hypermail/html-home/4-html/0057.html.

Eggs

1. F. B. Hu et al., "A prospective study of egg consumption and risk of cardiovascular disease in men and women," *JAMA*, 1999, 281: 1387–1394.
2. R. H. Knopp et. al., "A double-blind, randomized controlled trial of the effects of two eggs per day in moderately hypercholesterolemic and combined hyperlipidemic subjects taught the NCEP step 1 diet," *J Am College Nutrition*, 1997, 65: 1747–1764.
3. A. L. Gittleman, *Your Body Knows Best* (New York: Pocket Books, 1996), www.fatflush.com.
4. D. J. McNamara, "The impact of egg limitations on coronary heart disease risk: do the numbers add up?" *J Am Coll Nutr*, Oct 2000, 19(5 Suppl): 540S–548S.
5. G. Taubes, "The Soft Science of Dietary Fat," *Science*, March 30, 2001, 291: 2536–2545.
6. Gittleman.
7. D. Reuben, *Everything You Always Wanted to Know About Nutrition* (New York: Avon Books, 1978).
8. O. V. Garrison, *The Dictocrats—Our Unelected Rulers* (Chicago: Books For Today, Ltd., 1970).
9. *Ibid.*
10. Y. V. Yuan and D. D. Kitts, "Dietary fat source and cholesterol interactions alter plasma lipids and tissue susceptibility to oxidation in spontaneously hypertensive (SHR) and normotensive Wistar Kyoto (WKY) rats," *Mol Cell Biochem*, Mar 2002, 232(1-2): 33–47.
11. E. M. Cranton and J. P. Frackelton, "Free Radical Pathology in Age-Associated Diseases: Treatment with EDTA Chelation, Nutrition and Antioxidants," *Journal of Holistic Medicine*, Spring/Summer 1984, pp. 6–37.

12. E. Mindell, *Earl Mindell's Vitamin Bible* (New York: Warner Books, 1979).
13. Taubes.
14. USDA Foreign Agricultural Service, FASonline.
15. Reuben.
16. T. J. Moore, *Heart Failure* (New York: Simon and Schuster, 1989).
17. Uffe Ravnskov, *The Cholesterol Myths: Exposing the Fallacy That Saturated Fat and Cholesterol Cause Heart Disease* (Washington, D.C.: New Trends Publishing, Inc., 2000).
18. Robert Crayhon, *Nutrition Made Simple* (New York: M. Evans and Company, Inc., 1994).
19. Udo Erasmus, *Fats that Heal—Fats that Kill* (Burnaby, B.C., Canada: Alive Books, 1986).
20. Sally Fallon and Mary Enig, Ph.D., "Caustic Commentary," *Wise Traditions in Food, Farming and the Healing Arts,* Summer 2002, Vol. 3, No. 2, pp. 9–12.
21. Ravnskov.
22. D. Gaist et al., "Statins and risk of polyneuropathy: a case-control study," *Neurology,* May 14, 2002, 58 (9): 1333–1337.
23. A. Jula et al., "Effects of diet and simvastatin on serum lipids, insulin, and antioxidants in hypercholesterolemic men: a randomized controlled trial," *JAMA,* Feb 6, 2002, 287(5): 598–605.
24. T. B. Newman and S. B. Hulley, "Carcinogenicity of lipid-lowering drugs," *JAMA,* Jan 3, 1996, 275(1): 55–60.
25. R. Verdery, "Update in Women's Health" (Letters), *Annals of Internal Medicine,* Sept. 5, 2000, Vol. 133, No.5, p. 391.
26. K. Rizvi, J. P. Hampson, and J. N. Harvey, "Do lipid-lowering drugs cause erectile dysfunction? A systematic review," *Fam Pract,* Feb 2002, 19(1): 95–98.
27. ALLHAT officers and coordinators, "Major outcomes in moderately hypercholes-terolemic, hypertensive patients randomized to pravastatin vs usual care: The Antihypertensive and Lipid-Lowering Treatment to Prevent Heart Attack Trial (ALLHAT-LLT)," *JAMA,* Dec 18, 2002, 288(23): 2998–3007.
28. Ravnskov.
29. J. E. Bekelman, Y. Li, and P. Gross, "Scope and impact of financial conflicts of interest in biomedical research: a systematic review," *JAMA,* Jan 22–29, 2003, 289(4): 454–465.
30. Erasmus.
31. W. Sardi, "The Japanese Way of Health," *Health Journalist,* BillSardi.com/html-home/4-html/0057.html.

Plastics and Microwaves

1. *Male Reproductive Health and Environmental Chemicals with Estrogenic Effects,* The Danish Environmental Protection Agency, April 18, 1995.
2. Marla Cone, "River Pollution Study Finds Hormonal Defects in Fish," *The Los Angeles Times,* Sept. 22, 1998, p. 1.
3. E. Bauman, Ph.D., *Confronting Cancer In Our Community* (Cotati, California: Institute for Educational Therapy, 1998).
4. *Ibid.*
5. A. V. Krishnan et al., "Bisphenol-A: an estrogenic substance is released from polycarbonate flasks during autoclaving," *Endocrinology,* Jun 1993, 132 (6): 2279–2286.
6. H. Masuno et al., "Bisphenol A in combination with insulin can accelerate the conversion of 3T3-L1 fibroblasts to adipocytes," *J Lipid Res,* May 2002, 43(5): 676–684.
7. A. R. Singh, W. H. Lawrence, and J. Autian, "Maternal-fetal transfer of 14C-di-2-ethylhexyl pthalate and 14C-diethyl pthalate in rats," *J Pharm Sci,* Aug 1975, 64(8): 1347–1350.

8. L. A. Dostal, R. P. Weaver, and B. A. Schwetz, "Transfer of di(2-ethylhexyl) pthalate through rat milk and effects on milk consumption and the mammary gland," *Toxicol Appl Pharmacol*, Dec 1987, 91(3): 315–325.

9. D. C. Rice, "Parallels between attention deficit hyperactivity disorder and behavioral deficits produced by neurotoxic exposure in monkeys," *Environmental Health Perspectives*, 2000, 108(suppl 3): 405–408.

10. Sally Fallon and Mary Enig, Ph.D., "Response To Those Who Believe Soy Is Healthy," *Townsend Letter For Doctors and Patients*, April 2001, 213: 100–103.

11. H. Yoshida et al., "Effects of microwave cooking on the molecular species of pumpkin seed triacylglycerols," *Nutr Rep Int*, 1988, 37: 259–268.

12. M. G. Megahed, "Microwave roasting of peanuts: Effects on oil characteristics and composition," *Nahrung*, Aug 2001, 45(4): 255–257.

13. T. M. Vieira and M. A. Regitano-D'Arce, "Ultraviolet spectrophotometric evaluation of corn oil oxidative stability during microwave heating and oven test," *J Agric Food Chem*, Jun 1999, 47(6): 2203–2206.

14. C. Lai, *Pursuit of Life* (Soquel, CA: Lapis Lazuli Light, 1993).

15. Canton Bern Commercial Court (Mar. 19, 1993).

16. B. H. Blanc and H. U. Hertel, "Comparative Study about Food Prepared Conventionally and in the Microwave-Oven," *Raum&Zeit*, 1992, Vol. 3, No. 2, p. 43.

17. G. Lubec, C. Wolf, and B. Bartosch, "Aminoacid Isomerisation and Microwave Exposure," *Lancet*, 1989, 9: 1392–1393.

18. R. Quan et al., "Effects of microwave radiation on anti-infective factors in human milk," *Pediatrics*, 1992, 89(4): 667–669.

19. W. P. Kopp, "Effects of Microwaves on Humans," *J. Natural Science*, Apr.–Jun. 1998, Vol. 1. No. 1, pp. 42–43.

20. *Ibid.*

21. *Ibid.* (Editor's Note).

Vitamin C

1. H. Y. Huang et al., "Effects of vitamin C and vitamin E on in vivo lipid peroxidation: results of a randomized controlled trial," *Am J Clin Nutr*, Sep 2002, 76(3): 549–555.

2. M. Levine, C. Conry-Cantilena, Y. Wang, R. W. Welch, P. W. Washko, K. R. Dhariwal, J. B. Park, A. Lazarev, J. F. Graumlich, J. King, and L. R. Cantilena, "Vitamin C pharmacokinetics in healthy volunteers: evidence for a recommended dietary allowance," *Proc Natl Acad Sci* USA, Apr 16, 1996, 93(8): 3704–3709.

3. M. Levine, S. C. Rumsey, R. Daruwala et al., "Criteria and recommendations for vitamin C intake," *JAMA*, 1999, 281: 1415–1423.

4. I. D. Podmore, H. R. Griffiths, K. E. Herbert, N. Mistry, P. Mistry, and J. Lunec, "Vitamin C exhibits pro-oxidant properties," *Nature,* Apr 9, 1998, 392(6676): 559.

5. J. H. Dwyer, L. M. Nicholson, A. Shircore et al., "Vitamin C supplement intake and progression of carotid atherosclerosis," Los Angeles Atherosclerosis Study, #P82. (Presented at the American Heart Association's 40th Annual Conference on Cardiovascular Disease Epidemiology and Prevention, March 1–4, 2000.)

6. D. D. Waters et al., "Effects of hormone replacement therapy and antioxidant vitamin supplements on coronary atherosclerosis in postmenopausal women: a randomized controlled study," *JAMA*, Nov 20 2002, 288(19): 2432–2440.

7. S. Toyokuni, "Iron-induced carcinogenesis: the role of redox regulation," *Free Radic Biol Med*, 1996, 20(4): 553–566.

8. S. Johnson, "The possible crucial role of iron accumulation combined with low tryptophan, zinc and manganese in carcinogenesis," *Med Hypotheses*, Nov 2001, 57(5): 539–543.

9. D. Berg, M. Gerlach, M. B. Youdim, K. L. Double, L. Zecca, P. Riederer, and G. Becker "Brain iron pathways and their relevance to Parkinson's disease," *J Neurochem*, Oct 2001, 79(2): 225–236.

10. J. O. Kang, "Chronic iron overload and toxicity: clinical chemistry perspective," *Clin Lab Sci*, Summer 2001, 14(3): 209–219.

11. Robert Garrison and Elizabeth Somer, *The Nutrition Desk Reference* (New Canaan, CT: Keats Publishing, 1995).

12. S. F. Wong, B. Halliwell, R. Richmond, and W. R. Skowroneck. "The role of superoxide and hydroxyl radicals in the degradation of hyaluronic acid induced by metal ions and by ascorbic acid," *J Inorg Biochem*, Apr 1981, 14(2): 127–134.

13. H. Sakagami et al, "Apoptosis-inducing activity of vitamin C and vitamin K," *Cell. Mol. Biol.* (Noisy-le-grand), 2000, 46(1): 129–143.

14. S. H. Lee, T. Oe, and I. A. Blair. "Vitamin C-induced decomposition of lipid hydroperoxides to endogenous genotoxins," *Science*, Jun 15, 2001, 292(5524): 2083–2086.

15. "Lab study finds possible villainy in vitamin C pill," (08/13/2001, updated 05:43 PM ET), USATODAY.com.

16. D. B. Agus et al., "Vitamin C crosses the blood-brain barrier in the oxidized form through the glucose transporters," *J Clin Invest,* Dec 1, 1997, 100(11): 2842–2848.

17. A. Rehman et al., "The effects of iron and vitamin C co-supplementation on oxidative damage to DNA in healthy volunteers," *Biochem Biophys Res Commun*, May 8, 1998, 246(1): 293–298.

18. B. Halliwell, "Vitamin C and genotoxic stability," *Mutat Res*, Apr 2001, 475(1-2): 29–35.

19. S. H. Lee, T. Oe, and I. A. Blair.

20. B. Halliwell. "Vitamin C: antioxidant or pro-oxidant in vivo?" *Free Radic Res*, Nov 1996, 25(5): 439–454.

21. B. Halliwell, "Vitamin C: poison, prophylactic or panacea?" *Trends Biochem Sci*, Jul 1999, 24(7): 255–259.

22. *Ibid.*

23. A. Childs, C. Jacobs, T. Kaminski, B. Halliwell, and C. Leeuwenburgh. "Supplementation with vitamin C and N-acetyl-cysteine increases oxidative stress in humans after an acute muscle injury induced by eccentric exercise," *Free Radic Biol Med*, Sep 15, 2001, 31(6): 745–753.

24. Skye Lininger et al. *The Natural Pharmacy* (Sacramento, CA: Prima Health, 1998).

25. E. B. Finley and F. L. Cerklewski. "Influence of ascorbic acid supplementation on copper status in young adult men," *Am J Clin Nutr*, 1983, 37: 553–356.

26. C. R. Hansen, Jr., "Copper and zinc deficiencies in association with depression and neurological findings," *Biological Psychiatry*, 1983, 18(3): 395–401.

27. Thomas W. Johnson. "Copper—a 'Brain Food'," Grand Forks Human Nutrition Research Center (August 14,2001), http://www.gfhnrc.ars.usda.gov/News/nws9812a.htm.

28. Lininger.

29. Earl Mindell, *Vitamin Bible* (New York: Warner Books, 1979).

30. Garrison.

31. Robert Crayhon, *Nutrition Made Simple* (New York: M. Evans and Company, 1994).

32. "The Village of Long Life—Could Hyaluronic Acid Be an Anti-Aging Remedy?" (Nov. 2, 2000), ABC News.com.

33. R. M. Fink and E. Lengfelder. "Hyaluronic acid degradation by ascorbic acid and influence of iron," *Free Radic Res Commun*, 1987, 3(1-5): 85–92.

34. L. Vaillant and A. Callens, "Hormone replacement treatment and skin aging," *Therapie*, Jan–Feb 1996, 51(1): 67–70.

35. G. E. Goodman, "Prevention of lung cancer," *Crit Rev Oncol Hematol*, Mar 2000, 33(3): 187–197.

36. C. Marwick, "Trials reveal no benefit, possible harm of beta carotene and vitamin A for lung cancer prevention," *JAMA*, Feb 14, 1996, 275(6): 422–423.

37. M. Murata and S. Kawanishi, "Oxidative DNA damage by vitamin A and its derivative via superoxide generation," *J Biol Chem*, Jan 21, 2000, 275(3): 2003–2008.

38. Goodman.

39. "Lab study finds possible villainy in vitamin C pill" (08/13/2001, updated 05:43 PM ET), USATODAY.com.

Food Irradiation

1. Dr. Dean Edell, "Eating Right," *Washington Post*, March 28, 2000, p. Z11.

2. Donald B. Louria, "Zapping the food supply," *Bulletin of the Atomic Scientists*, June 1990, Vol. 46, No. 5, pp. ?.

3. *Ibid.*

4. C. Bhaskaram and G. Sadasivan, "Effects of Feeding Irradiated Wheat to Malnourished Children," *American Journal of Clinical Nutrition*, 1975, Vol. 28, No. 2, pp. 130–35.

5. P. Maier et al., "Cell-Cycle and Ploidy Analysis in Bone Marrow and Liver Cells of Rats after Long-Term Consumption of Irradiated Wheat," *Food Chem Toxicol*, Jun 1993; 31(6): 395–405.

6. "Potential Health Hazards of Food Irradiation," Verbatim Excerpts from Expert Testimony (June 19, 1987), U.S. Congressional Hearings into Food Irradiation, House Committee on Energy and Commerce, Subcommittee on Health and the Environment.

7. Udo Erasmus, *Fats that Heal—Fats that Kill* (Burnaby, B.C., Canada: Alive Books, 1986).

8. Public Citizen (articles, links, references for food irradiation), http://www.citizen.org/cmep/foodsafety/food_irrad/.

9. W. W. Au, "Expert Affidavit on Safety Issues of Irradiated Food for School Children," www.citizen.org/documents/williamauaffidavit.pdf.

10. "FDA Ignoring Evidence that New Chemicals created in irradiated food could be harmful" (Nov. 29, 2001), The Center for Food Safety. Press release by Public Citizen.

11. Au.

12. http://www.mercola.com/article/Diet/irradiated/irradiated_research.htm.

13. John Gofman, Letter to Margaret Seckler, Secretary of U.S. Department of Health and Human Services, February 28, 1984.

14. Louria.

15. E. Wierbicki et al., "Ionizing Energy in Food Processing and Pest Control, Part 1" (July 1986), Council for Agricultural Science and Technology, Ames, Iowa.

16. "Irradiation compounds vitamin loss from cooking," ARS Report, *Food Chemical News*, Nov. 10, 1986, p. 42.

17. H. Julius, *Irradiated Foods*, Friends of the Earth, 1999, http://www.mindfully.org/Food/Irradiated-Food-Julius-FOE1999.htm.

18. Samuel S. Epstein and Wenonah Hauter, "Preventing Pathogenic Food Poisoning: Sanitation not Irradiation," *International Journal of Health Services*, 2001, Vol. 31, No. 1, pp. 187–192.

19. "Arsenic in Drinking Water: 2001 Update" (October 4, 2001), testimony of Robert A. Goyer, Professor Emeritus University of Western Ontario and Chair, Subcommittee to Update the 1999 Arsenic in Drinking Water Report, Board on Environmental Studies and Toxicology, National Research Council, before the House Science Committee, U.S. House of Representatives.

20. "EPA Withdraws Arsenic in Tap Water Rules," Clean Water Action, Mar. 21, 2001.
21. "EPA Announces Arsenic Standard for Drinking Water of 10 Parts per Billion" (10/31/2001), EPA Headquarters Press Release.
22. Louria.
23. K. Terry, "Why is DoE for Food Irradiation?" *The Nation,* Feb. 7, 1987, pp. 142–156.
24. "Administration Proposal to Serve Irradiated Beef to School Children Poses Cancer, Genetic and Other Risks warns Samuel S. Epstein" (April 8, 2001), Press release, Chicago.
25. "Bush School Lunch Proposal: Yet Another Favor to Special Interests That Funded Campaign" (April 15, 2001). Press release by Public Citizen. Common Dreams Newscenter (www.commondreams.org/news2001/0405-04.htm).

Vegetarianism

1. Sally Fallon with Mary Enig, Ph.D., *Nourishing Traditions* (Washington, D.C.: New Trends Publishing, Inc., 1999, 2001).
2. *Ibid.*
3. Robert Aitken, *The Mind of Clover* (San Francisco: North Point Press, 1984).
4. Peter Tompkins and Christopher Bird, *The Secret Life of Plants* (New York: Avon Books, 1973).
5. Charles Eisenstein, "The Ethics of Eating Meat: A Radical View," *Wise Traditions in Food, Farming and the Healing Arts,* Vol. 3, No. 2. (Summer 2002), pp. 21–25.
6. Fallon and Enig.
7. Robert M. Crayhon, *The Carnitine Miracle* (New York: M. Evans and Company, Inc., 1998).
8. Fallon and Enig.
9. Stephen Byrnes, "Myths and Truths About Vegetarianism," *Townsend Letter for Doctors and Patients,* July 2000, pp. 72–81.
10. E. A. Enas, "Coronary artery disease epidemic in Indians: a cause for alarm and call for action," *J Indian Med Assoc,* Nov 2000, 98 (11): 694–695, 697–702.
11. Fallon and Enig.
12. J. Sabate, "Nut consumption, vegetarian diets, ischemic heart disease risk, and all-cause mortality: evidence from epidemiologic studies," *Am J Clin Nutr,* Sep 1999; 70(3 Suppl): 500S–503S.
13. Earl Mindell, *Vitamin Bible* (New York: Warner Books, 1979).
14. T. Kuhne, R. Bubl, and R. Baumgartner, "Maternal vegan diet causing a serious infantile neurological disorder due to vitamin B12 deficiency," *Eur J Pediatric,* Jan 1991, 150(3): 205–208.
15. F. Renault, P. Verstichel, J. P. Ploussard, and J. Costil, "Neuropathy in two cobalamin [vitamin B12]-deficient breast-fed infants of vegetarian mothers," *Muscle Nerve,* Feb 1999, 22(2): 252–254.
16. M. Krajcovicova-Kudlackova et al., "Homocysteine levels in vegetarians versus omnivores," *Ann Nutr Meta,* 2000, 44(3): 135–138.
17. Mindell.
18. Byrnes.
19. T. J. A. Key, M. Thorogood, J. Keenan, and A. Long, "Raised thyroid stimulating hormone associated with kelp intake in British vegan men," *J Hum Nutr Diet,* 1992, 5:323–326.
20. M. Labib, R. Gama, J. Wright, V. Marks, and D. Robins, "Dietary maladvice as a cause of hypothyroidism and short stature," *BMJ,* Jan 28, 1989, 298(6668): 232–233.
21. Fallon and Enig.

22. *Ibid.*

23. *Ibid.*

24. *Ibid.*

25. *Ibid.*

26. T. A. Outila, M. U. Karkkainen, R. H. Seppanen, and C. J. Lamberg-Allardt, "Dietary intake of vitamin D in premenopausal, healthy vegans was insufficient to maintain concentrations of serum 25-hydroxyvitamin D and intact parathyroid hormone within normal ranges during the winter in Finland," *J Am Diet Assoc,* Apr 2000, 100(4): 434–441.

27. J. F. Chiu et al., "Long-term vegetarian diet and bone mineral density in postmenopausal Taiwanese women," *Calcif Tissue Int,* Mar 1997, 60(3): 245–249.

28. L. Bostman and O. Bostman, "Acute osteoporosis in a breast-feeding vegetarian woman," *Duodecim,* 1988, 104(12): 937–940.

29. B. Sandstrom, H. Andersson, B. Kivisto, and A. S. Sandberg, "Apparent small intestinal absorption of nitrogen and minerals from soy and meat-protein-based diets. A study on human ileostomy subjects," *J Nutr,* Nov 1986, 116(11): 2209–2218.

30. R. F. Hurrell, M. A. Juillerat, M. B. Reddy, S. R. Lynch, S. A. Dassenko, and J. D. Cook, "Soy protein, phytate, and iron absorption in humans," *Am J Clin Nutr,* Sep 1992, 56(3): 573–578.

31. F. Perez-Llamas, M. Garaulet, J. A. Martinez, J. F. Marin, E. Larque, and S. Zamora, "Influence of dietary protein type and iron source on the absorption of amino acids and minerals," *J Physiol Biochem,* Dec 2001, 57(4): 321–328.

32. http://www.soyonlineservice.co.nz/soytox.htm.

33. I. E. Liener, "Implications of antinutritional components in soybean food," *Crit Rev Food Sci Nutr,* 1994, 34(1): 31–67.

34. Crayhon.

35. *Ibid*

36. Fallon and Enig.

37. *Ibid.*

38. *Ibid.*

39. E. M. Lau, T. Kwok, J. Woo, and S. C. Ho, "Bone mineral density in Chinese elderly female vegetarians, vegans, lacto-vegetarians and omnivores," *Eur J Clin Nutr,* Jan 1998; 52(1): 60–64.

40. S. T. Reddy, C. Y. Wang, K. Sakhaee, L. Brinkley, amd C. Y. Pak, "Effect of low-carbohydrate high-protein diets on acid-base balance, stone-forming propensity, and calcium metabolism," *Am J Kidney Dis,* Aug 2002, 40(2): 265–274.

41. D. R. Jacobs, Jr.; K. A. Meyer; L. H. Kushi; and A. R. Folsom; "Whole-grain intake may reduce the risk of ischemic heart disease death in postmenopausal women: the Iowa Women's Health Stud;," *Am J Clin Nutr;* Aug 1998; 68(2): 248–257.

42. Fallon and Enig.

43. Crayhon.

44. L. Cordain, S. B. Eaton, J. Brand Miller, N. Mann, and K. Hill, "The paradoxical nature of hunter-gatherer diets: Meat based, yet non-atherogenic," *Eur J Clin Nutr,* 2002, 56(suppl 1): S42–S52.

45. David L. Freed, "Do dietary lectins cause disease?" *BMJ,* Apr 17, 1999, 318: 1023–1024.

46. Crayhon.

47. K. North and J. Golding, "A maternal vegetarian diet in pregnancy is associated with hypospadias" (The ALSPAC Study Team, Avon Longitudinal Study of Pregnancy and Childhood), *BJU Int,* Jan 2000, 85(1): 107–113.

48. Marian Burros, "Eating Well—Anti-Organic, and Flawed," *New York Times,* February 17, 1999, p. 5.

49. Nancy Creamer, "CDC has never compared *E. coli* risks of organic, traditional food," College of Agriculture and Life Sciences, North Carolina State University, Raleigh, *VEG-I-NEWS*, February 1999 (http://ipm.ncsu.edu/vegetables/veginews/veginw14.htm).

50. Virginia Worthington, "Effect of Agricultural Methods on Nutritional Quality: A Comparison of Organic with Conventional Crops," *Alternative Therapies in Health and Medicine*, Jan 1998, Vol. 4, No. 1, pp. 58–69.

51. *Ibid.*

52. Mark Purdey, "The (Vegan Ecological) Wasteland," *Price-Pottenger Nutrition Foundation Health Journal*, 1999, Vol. 22, No. 4, pp. ?.

53. Anthony R. Measham and Meera Chatterjee, "Wasting Away—The Crisis of Malnutrition in India," *World Bank Report* (World Bank Group, Washington, D.C.), May 1999.

54. Fallon and Enig.

55. Purdey.

The Best Diet

1. Alan Gaby book review of *The Blood Type Diet* in *Nutrition and Healing Newsletter*, (Phoenix, AZ, January 1998), p. 7.

2. Walter Willett, *Eat, Drink, and Be Healthy* (New York: Simon & Schuster, 2001).

3. Larry Dossey, "The 'Eating-Papers' and Other Curious Aspects of Nutrition," *Alternative Therapies in Health and Medicine*, Nov. 1998, Vol. 4, No. 6, pp. 11–16, 99–104.

4. *Ibid.*

5. Robert Crayhon, *The Carnitine Miracle* (New York: Evans and Company, 1998).

6. P. Roberts, "The New Food Anxiety," *Psychol Today*, Mar./Apr. 1998: 30ff.

7. Marc David, *Nourishing Wisdom* (New York: Bell Tower, 1991).

8. Crayhon.

9. S. Eaton, S. Boyd et al., *The Paleolithic Prescription* (New York: Harper & Row Publishers, 1988).

10. Elson M. Haas, *Staying Healthy with Nutrition: The Complete Guide to Diet and Nutritional Medicine* (Berkeley: Ten Speed Press, 1990).

11. Crayhon.

Index

Author's Endnote: A Teacher and Parent's Perspective

Americans consume 25 percent of their calories in the form of cookies, chips, candy, cakes, ice cream, and soda; and for one in every three Americans, 45 percent of their calories come from these "foods." Is it any wonder, then, why heart disease, obesity, and diabetes are so common today? When you add to this situation the thyroid-inhibiting effects of fluoridated water and unfermented soy products, we have nothing less than a disaster.

Even sadder is the pronounced effect that *trans* fats, refined flour, and sugary foods are having on our children. In addition, health-conscious adults who attempt to get their children to eat a "politically correct" low-fat diet usually make the problem worse.

I have been a teacher of children for nearly thirty years. During those years, I have witnessed growing rates of obesity and hyperactivity, and have seen the quality of lunches go from bad to worse. Attempting to play a small part in stemming the tide of this form of child abuse, in recent years I have worked with a privately funded group of educators who go into public schools to instruct youngsters in the areas of physiology, drug prevention, and nutrition. In the area of nutrition, often we are teaching the children to go home and educate their parents.

The job is not easy. We are working with children who, in many cases, are already struggling with learning disabilities as well as with endocrine and thyroid disruption that may have been caused by soy formulas fed to them as infants. Many are impaired by a lack of essential fats in their current diets. Many cannot concentrate or listen well. And a good number of them are unable to learn. A surprising number of children come to school without eating breakfast. For lunch, their parents provide food that consists of the most convenient things to throw into a bag: chips, boxed fruit punches, processed cheeses, colas, fruit "leather," candy bars, and hastily made sandwiches on white bread.

If they eat at the school cafeteria, they may have access to soda vending machines and to fast-food-quality fare or, in the case of some politically correct food providers, be subject to the dangers and deficiencies of soy and low-fat products that lack healthy fats for healthy brains. In many cases, children have been conditioned to eat only the fried or processed foods; they may eat a side dish of fruit cocktail, but the fresh apple or orange served to them winds up in the trash.

The outlook is not good for the health of our children. Children whose diets are low in important nutrients also face the specter of acne, early osteoporosis, dental irregularities, and problems with brain chemistry, which can lead to violent behavior. Aware of the health problems facing our children today, government agencies like the USDA claim they are doing a service by developing lower-fat meals for school lunches (in addition to pushing for the use of irradiated beef in school lunches).

According to Dr. Mary Enig of the Weston A. Price Foundation, these lower-fat diets are actually causing some of the very problems they were designed to prevent. She adds, "Children need a diet rich in traditional fats in order to achieve optimum growth and development, as well as protection from heart disease later in life."

What can we do as adults to protect our children from chronic diseases that are the result of the highly refined American diet, food irradiation, bovine growth hormone, and the dangers of aspartame and fluoridation (with its accompanying levels of brain-damaging lead)? What can we do to help raise a generation of children whose level of physical and mental health will promote self-esteem and the ability to be happy and to succeed in this world? First, we can educate ourselves. And then we can become active in fighting to change those political and corporate interests that act to undermine the health of all Americans in the name of profit.

I have found the Weston A. Price Foundation to be of help in this cause. According to their Web site (w.w.w.westonaprice.org), "The Foundation is dedicated to restoring nutrient-dense foods to the human diet through education, research, and activism. It supports a number of movements that contribute to this objective, including accurate nutrition instruction, organic and biodynamic farming, pasture-feeding of livestock, community-supported farms, honest and informative labeling, prepared parenting and nurturing therapies. Specific goals include establishment of universal access to clean, certified raw milk and a ban on the use of soy formula for infants."

When we become activists and make the necessary changes, the results are often phenomenal. A case in point is what happened in 1997 at Central Alternative High School in Appleton, Wisconsin. It had been a school out of control with a high number of discipline problems. Some students even carried weapons.

At that time a private group called Natural Ovens initiated a truly healthy lunch program. Access to soda, candy, chips, and chemically processed food items was prohibited. No more fried, highly processed, or sugary foods. No more vending machines and packed lunches. Instead, students were served salads, fruits and vegetables, pure water, and baked meats, as well as soups, stews, and entrees made from scratch. In addition, the kids gained knowledge of the role a healthy diet plays in an improved quality of life, and gained an understanding of how good nutrition supports a healthy brain and how proper eating can prevent certain life-threatening diseases.

A few years later, the environment at Central Alternative High showed an enormous change. As reported in the Feingold Association's newsletter "Pure Facts" (http://www.lauralee.com/news/healthylunch.htm): "Grades are up, truancy is no longer a problem, arguments are rare, and teachers are able to spend their time teaching." One teacher stated, "I don't have to deal with daily discipline issues—I don't have disruptions in class or the difficulties with student behavior I experienced before we started the food program." In addition, there were no longer any drop outs or expelled students, and none carried weapons. There were no suicides and no students found to be using drugs.

This sounds something like a miracle. But perhaps traditional, unprocessed, nutrient-dense foods should always be considered miraculous by virtue of their ability to heal and strengthen both body and mind. As evidenced by the Wisconsin teenagers, it's never too late to make smart, dietary changes that are not based on what food-industry propaganda tells us, but rather on the types of food which have sustained cultures for thousands of years. We owe it to our children. We owe it to ourselves.

Michael Barbee
December, 2003

RESOURCE APPENDIX

The following is a list of information and activism resources.

Aspartame Truth, www.aspartametruth.com
If you've been consuming aspartame thinking you have no problems as a result, chances are you have symptoms that you don't associate with aspartame. If you consume aspartame and have obvious health problems that no doctor has been able to help you with—e.g., arthritis pain, vision problems—I strongly recommend you take the "aspartame challenge": Stop consuming all aspartame products for at least a few weeks and see if your symptoms are alleviated. The site has links to other sites as well as to FDA files on aspartame.

Bovine Growth Hormone Site, www.foxbghsuit.com
Here you will find behind-the-scenes details about how a large share of America's milk supply has quietly become adulterated from the effects of the synthetic bovine growth hormone (BGH) secretly injected into cows, and how pressure from the hormone maker, Monsanto, led Fox TV to fire two of its award-winning reporters, suppressing what they discovered but were never allowed to broadcast.

Campaign for Raw Milk, www.realmilk.com

CETOS, www.cetos.org
An organization committed to protecting vulnerable populations from harmful toxicants, and to assuring a toxic-free world for our children and our children's children. CETOS books on bioengineering: *Against the Grain* (Common Courage Press, 1998), *Engineering the Farm* (Island Press, 2002), and *Cutting DNA* (Common Courage Press, 2003).

Cholesterol Myths, www.ravnskov.nu/cholesterol.htm

Citizens For Health, www.citizens.org
Works to expand your healthcare choices because you have a right to: Choose your physicians, including naturopaths, homeopaths, chiropractors, acupuncturists, and others providing alternative therapies; choose treatments, including vitamin supplements, herbs, homeopathy, and other nonconventional modalities; purchase vitamins, herbs, and other supplements easily and in the dosages you require; obtain water that is free of toxins and harmful chemicals; eat natural foods grown and prepared without pesticides, hormones, or antibiotics; be fully informed if foods for purchase have been irradiated or genetically engineered; and be fully informed on issues affecting your freedom of choice.

Feingold Association, www.feingold.org
An organization of families and professionals, the Feingold® Association of the United States is dedicated to helping children and adults apply proven dietary techniques for better behavior, learning, and health.

Food First, www.foodfirst.org
A member-supported, nonprofit, people's think tank and education-for-action center for re-claiming our rights to safe, sustainable food production. Great action/educational newsletter. Focuses on Genetic Engineering.

Food Integrity Resources Site, www.foodintegrity.com
Excellent source of independent information, commentary, news, and articles about our food and water supply, and links to other reviewed sites. Compiled by Vital Health Publishing and Michael Barbee.

Greenpeace True Food Network, www.truefoodnow.org, 415-512-9024
A free service to connect consumers who want to take action to end the use of genetically engineered (GE) ingredients in our foods. The Network calls on food companies, like Safeway and Shaw's, to stop using GE ingredients in our food. By joining you will be connected to thousands of other consumers across the country who are saying no to the biotech industry's secret experiment with our food supply and saying yes to sustainably grown food.

Institute of Science in Society, www.i-sis.org.uk
Provides both frightful and inspiring news about the latest science on genetically modified foods and environmental toxins by leading scientists, news of the UK's fight to stop genetically modified foods from taking over, a free newsletter, alerts. Founder Mae-Wan Ho's book, *GMO Free* is published by Vital Health Publishing. Available as PDF online.

Linus Pauling Institute, lpi.oregonstate.edu/
The Institute functions from the basic premise that an optimum diet is the key to optimum health. Our mission is to determine the function and role of micronutrients, vitamins, and phytochemicals in promoting optimum health and preventing and treating disease, and to determine the role of oxidative and nitrative stress and antioxidants in human health.

Mercola, www.mercola.com
Sign up for a newsletter from Dr. Mercola, author of "The No Grain Diet."

Paleolithic Diet Page, www.panix.com/~paleodiet/
Web resource page for information on the caveman diet.

Power Health, www.powerhealth.net
Articles here offer good information on recent findings on whole foods and natural health.

Practical Hippie, www.practicalhippie.com/irradiation.htm
This site features information on health, environmental, and social issues from an independent researcher/activist and professionally trained librarian. Food irradiation is one such topic.

Public Citizen, www.citizen.org
A national, nonprofit consumer advocacy organization founded by Ralph Nader in 1971 to represent consumer interests in Congress, the executive branch, and the courts. Fights for openness and democratic accountability in government, for the right of consumers to seek redress in the courts; for clean, safe, and sustainable energy sources; for social and economic justice in trade policies; for strong health, safety, and environmental protections; and for safe, effective, and affordable prescription drugs and healthcare.

Pure Food, www.pure-food.com
The intent of this Web site is to educate and raise awareness regarding the degradation of our food supply and our individual liberties by big government and big business and the public relations ploys designed to hide the truth.

Soy Online, www.soyonlineservice.co.nz/
Incredible information on the realities of the soy industry: who's behind the propaganda, latest news, and what you can do about it.

Udo Erasmus' Web Site, www.udoerasmus.com/firstscreen.htm
Shares articles about the importance of essential fatty acids and information about the failings of the Food Pyramid recommended by the USDA.

Weston A. Price Foundation, www.westonaprice.org
A nonprofit, tax-exempt charity founded in 1999 to disseminate the research of nutrition pioneer Dr. Weston Price, whose studies of isolated, nonindustrialized peoples established the parameters of human health and determined the optimum characteristics of human diets. The Foundation is dedicated to restoring nutrient-dense foods to the human diet through education, research, and activism.

What Doctors Don't Tell You, www.wddty.com
Helps you make an informed decision by giving you the facts you won't read anywhere else. "What Doctors Don't Tell You," the monthly newsletter and information service, reveals the hidden truth about medicine. Subscribe online.

FLUORIDE

Australian Fluoridation News, www.glenwalker.net
Artificial fluoridation is water pollution! If you don't fight it, you won't stop it!

Citizens for Safe Drinking Water, www.Keepers-of-the-Well.org
Exposes the hidden truths about fluoridation, who knows about it already, and how to force action.

Fluoridation.com, www.fluoridation.com

Fluoride Action Network, www.fluoridealert.org
An international coalition working to end water fluoridation and alert the public to fluoride's health and environmental risks.

National Pure Water Association, www.npwa.freeserve.co.uk/fluoride.html
Read the research that has demonstrated that fluoride has many serious adverse effects, such as cancer, osteoporosis, dental fluorosis, genetic abnormalities and brain damage in children.

NY State Coalition Opposed to Fluoridation, www.orgsites.com/ny/nyscof

Parents of Fluoride Poisoned Children, http://64.177.90.157/pfpc/index.html
This site is mainly about fluoride poisoning that occurs in our children—from any and all sources, whether soy products, toothpaste or other oral dental products, fluoride tablets, tea, and air pollution.

Stop Fluoridation USA, www.rvi.net/~fluoride/

If You Enjoyed *Politically Incorrect Nutrition,* Check Out These Other Vital Health Titles!

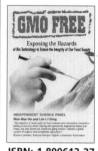
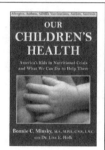
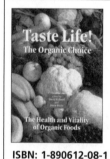

Vital Health Publishing
PO Box 152, Ridgefield, CT 06877
info@vitalhealthbooks.com
203-894-1882
www.vitalhealthbooks.com
To Order: 877-VIT-BOOKS